Intermittent Fasting

The Complete Guide to Lose Weight, Heal Your Body & Live a Healthy Life

CHRISTOPHER COLLINS

Table of Contents

Introduction: What is Wrong With Our Diet?

There is a huge disconnect between us and the food that we eat. The obesity epidemic is an ever-growing problem that we face in society today. The standard American diet contains approximately 60% of carbohydrates, which is an outstanding imbalance, and is one of the main causes of obesity today. However, if you follow intermittent fasting religiously, you will find yourself consuming less than half of this amount in carbohydrates.

We live in a society where our lives seem to revolve around food and staying at home in front of our computers or television; we don't go outside to enjoy nature or the park with our kids. We have our noses buried in work, and when we're not working, we bury ourselves in food. There are restaurants and fast food joints around every corner of the civilized world reminding us it's time to eat.

We have no sense of limiting ourselves in any area of our lives, especially with food. The food industry makes it all too easy to overeat with upgraded sizes and promotions that make us feel like we deserve the reward of enjoying our favorite greasy burger — at 3am. With the convenience of food revolving around our lives in the form of 24-hour grocery stores and fast food restaurants, it's hard to sit back and think about how we should put a stop to this behavior.

We can see the impact of food when we look at our wallets, and the latest statistics for 2019 might shock you; the average American person — not household — will spend about $7,700 a year on food and eating out, which equates to about $641 per month or $160 per week! Food is the most expensive item in any budget behind housing and transportation costs. Once you figure out your monthly budget, it will amaze you how much money goes towards feeding ourselves. Because you normally wouldn't make one large payment a month, such as your rent, mortgage or car payment, food expenses go under the radar. Only those who stick to a close budget know the costs they are dishing out on food[47].

Why would we want to give up on something that fills us with so much pleasure and that we could get just by jumping in our car and driving around the corner?

Because we want something better for ourselves. When we see the outcome of our terrible choices and observe the awful effects, it is when we become active in fixing the problem. We notice when our health becomes a real problem: when we can no longer run and play with our kids like we used to, or we can't climb the stairs without stopping to catch our breath. Maybe it's gone too far and a major disease has built up in your body, and you have to face the dire consequences of your choices.

Because of our ill relationship and downright disrespect of food, we are seeing major health problems skyrocket in our society. Obesity rates are the highest statistics the National Health and Nutrition Examination Survey (NHANES) has ever reported: nearly 40% of adults and 18% of children are obese[14]; diabetes affects over 425 million adults throughout the world[17]; cardiovascular disease (CVD) is the leading cause of death within the United States with over 800,000 deaths a year[64]; and cancer is the next big disease which causes over 600,000 deaths each year with 1.7 million people being diagnosed just this year[57]. And these are just the heavy hitters.

Whatever your personal case may be, there is always hope. Every day, you can make choices about everything that you do. You can continue to wallow in what your life and health have become or you can work towards changing it. We have all seen the shows on television where people who were massively overweight run around in their bikinis in Cancun, or the man who beat cancer because he took control of his life and choices into his own hands. We all know that it's possible, and the possibilities can be made a reality with intermittent fasting.

There can be a lot of confusion with how intermittent fasting works. Is it for weight loss? Yes, weight loss is a large component of this lifestyle. However, there are so many more benefits that we can derive from following intermittent fasting methods. Through this book, you will realize the possibilities that can come from fasting. It's a complex subject, yet it can be simple for people who are determined to learn and understand it. Millions of people have seen actual, long-term results in which they can keep the weight off.

Why? Because they have changed their relationship with food. It is no longer a go-to when they are bored or are having a rough day. Food is no longer a celebratory thing that they indulge upon. They are no longer a slave to their addictions, and most of all, they love what they look and feel like after they have reached their personal weight goals. They now respect food and the nourishment it can give to their bodies, and they love themselves enough to improve their lives.

Even though there is a small group of people whom doctors and specialists do not recommend follow any intermittent fasting methods, most people can follow this plan on their own. For those who are trying to overcome an illness, you should work with your doctor to reach your personal health goals because your body will be experiencing many dramatic changes.

It is not always going to be an easy process, but is it really worth having if it was just given to you? Your goals will need to be solid in your mind to remind you of the amazing reward you are working toward, and you will need to stay strong and committed in order to reach those goals.

The love you have for yourself will drive you through your intermittent fasting journey to realize all the possible benefits you could receive. The number one goal is weight loss; however, there are several other benefits that people see while using intermittent fasting methods. You will:

- Have more energy
- Feel more aware and clear-headed
- Lower cholesterol, blood pressure, and risks for stroke and heart disease
- Feel less hungry and learning to eat the correct amount of food required for your body
- Reduce your insulin sensitivity, high glucose levels, and medications for diabetes
- Lower your chance for neurological disorders such as Alzheimer's disease and Parkinson's disease
- Improve your memory and learning capabilities
- And many more!

There have been numerous studies done over the course of the last few decades on the effectiveness of intermittent fasting and the wellbeing of a person, and several of these studies have found positive results on humans and animals alike. The results are astounding from a scientific and personal standpoint. You will find out more about the science as you continue to read through this book.

You have taken the first step in changing your life through intermittent fasting just by purchasing this book and doing so shows that your initiative is strong. It is a promise that once you understand the mechanisms and proof behind intermittent fasting that you will see real physical changes in yourself. Usually, people will notice major changes within the first few weeks. For others, it may take a little longer. However, if you stick with it, you will see positive results of intermittent fasting.

There's nothing to wait for. You have the power to change your life starting today, and you will begin to see the world in a whole new light when you succeed with the intermittent fasting program and methods. You will learn how to incorporate all the aspects of this lifestyle into your life, and you will notice the impactful changes occurring in your life as a result.

So let us get started on working towards achieving success in your personal goals!

Part One: Overview of Intermittent Fasting

Chapter 1: What is Fasting?

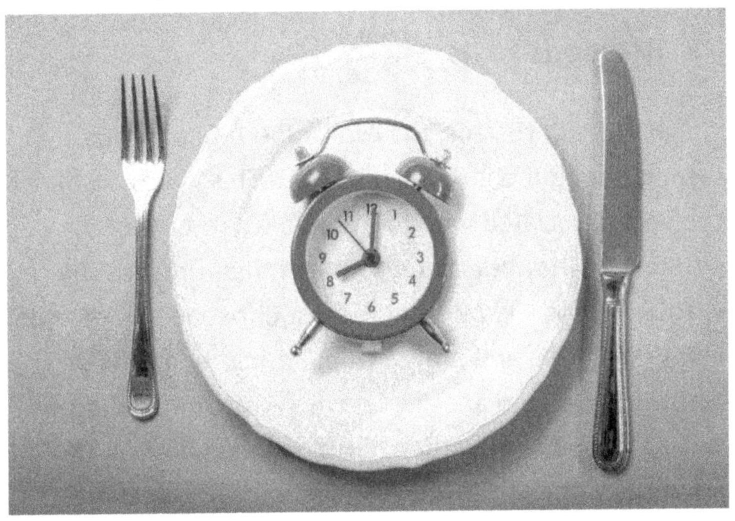

Human civilization has practiced fasting throughout all of history. The first people who practiced fasting were the ancient hunter-gatherers, as they had to find their food rather than have the convenience of going out to buy the food as we can today. Because they had to search, they were not always successful and as a result, they would sometimes go without food for stretches at a time. As their bodies evolved, they reached a point where they could function without eating constantly.

Beyond the history of the hunter-gatherers, religious communities that practiced Buddhism, Hinduism, Christianity, Judaism, and Islam also incorporated fasting into their culture.

Religious Fasts

For the Christians, they will adhere to a form of fasting during the forty days of Lent. This was the time of the year associated with Easter and was a type of penitence. They associated this length of time fasting with Jesus and the prophet Moses. Christians believe that self-humiliation and prayer would bring themselves closer to God, and ancient Christians meant for the fasting period to be a time of reflection and a test to strengthen the mind, body, and spirit.

In Judaism, Day of Atonement, known as *Yom Kippur,* is the day that Jews would be cleansed of their sins. The name derives from Hebrew for "self-denial." Yom Kippur falls eight days after the start of the Jewish New Year, *Rosh Hashanah,* and they believed that on their New Year, God writes the names of all the Jews into the "books" along with their judgment, and this opportunity would come on *Yom Kippur.* They conduct the Day of Atonement for a full 25 hours, beginning at sunset the night before *Yom Kippur* and concluded in the evening the next night.

They conduct a hard fast by drinking no fluids or only eating during a specified time frame. In addition, it is forbidden for them to wear leather shoes, bathe themselves, have sexual relations, or put lotion on their skin.

Jainism, Buddhism, and Hinduism all practice Fasting in the East. Both Jainism and Buddhism came into being around 500 BC in India, both as branches of Hinduism. Because they were born out of a single religious thought, they are similar in their fasting practices.

The purpose of fasting in all these religions is for spiritual gains. The result is a parallel connection between the body and the soul, a balance that is imperative in their way of life. They also fast to build their self-discipline. It is a belief of the Hindus that food exists to gratify the senses; if they were to take away the gratification from the senses, it would force the self to contemplate.

Fasts are associated with moon cycles, religious practices, festivals, and rituals. They are also related to the specific form of God they worship, which will coincide with the specific day of the week they must fast. Distinct major festivals for the Hindus are *Shivratri*, *Karwa Chauth*, and *Navaratri* where they fast.

In the East, a fast can mean abstaining from a particular food or spice, or only eating fruit on a certain day. Fasting can even garner respect, as in the case with Gandhi and his performing fasts as a form of peaceful protest.

In the Islam faith, they have reformed fasting to an art. There are several purposes and rules surrounding their fasting and it has become a natural way of life. They treat it as a way to become enlightened about their self-purification. They focus on adhering to the hours of the fast by eating a traditional meal known as the *sehri* just before the fast is to begin, up to the time of the morning prayer.

Muslims base their fasts solely on the lunar calendar. In this way, it makes it easier for all Muslims to start at the same time, no matter how distant they are from civilization.

Other Types of Fasts

There are other types of fasting which include the following:

Cleansing Fast: A period of fasting followed by a diet of water, fruit juices, vegetables, and fruit.

Diagnostic Fast: A fast required before medical procedures such as blood tests.

Full Fast: A fast where the individual does not allow for any food or fluid into the body.

Juice Fast: A set period set aside for fasting from solid foods; the individual may only consume vegetable and fruit juice.

Liquid Protein Fast: A shake fast; the individual abstains from caloric drinks and solid food. The shakes are full of minerals, vitamins, and a large amount of protein.

Regular Fast: The individual does not consume food; however, they may still drink fluids with no calories.

Partial Fast: The individual abstains from a type of food or drink for religious or health reasons; may include meat, dairy products, or wheat. Occurs for a specific amount of time.

Sexual Fast: Specific period where one abstains from sexual activity in all forms.

Water Fast: For a set period, the individual may only consume water. This is a detoxification fast.

Chapter Summary

- The history of fasting goes back several centuries. When the hunter-gatherers could not find food, their bodies would naturally go through the fasting process.
- Fasting is commonly used for spiritual purposes. Middle Eastern and Eastern religions all perform some kind of fasting.
- There are several fasts that an individual can incorporate such as abstaining from sexual activity, solid foods, or even specific foods like meat or wheat.

In the next chapter, we will go over the basics of intermittent fasting and the benefits associated with following the intermittent fasting methods.

Chapter 2: What is Intermittent Fasting, and Why is it Right for You?

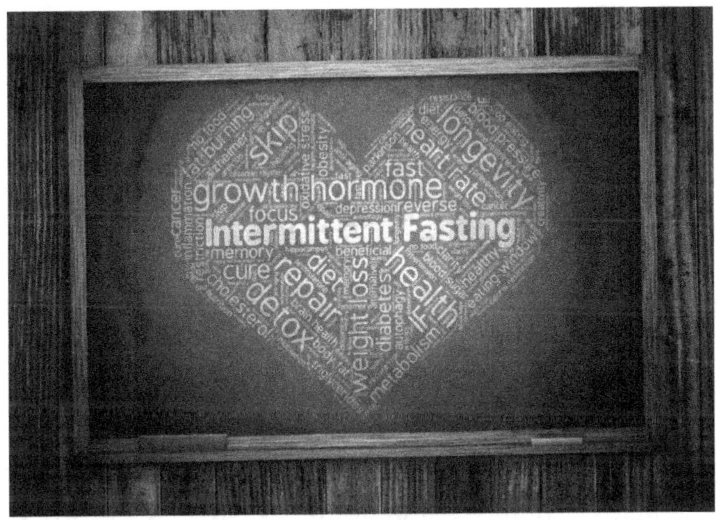

With intermittent fasting, there exists much confusion and myths surrounding what it entails. The basis of intermittent fasting is switching back and forth between eating and fasting. An **eating window** is when an individual can eat a normal amount of food over a short period.

There are no rigid diet rules, as intermittent fasting has more to do with the times at which an individual eats. Because of this, intermittent fasting is more like an eating pattern rather than a diet.

Once you can follow the concept of intermittent fasting, you will be on the fast track toward a healthy weight loss.

The Health Benefits of Intermittent Fasting

You can enjoy several benefits of intermittent fasting while following its process. One benefit is how it can help those suffering from diabetes, as it can enhance insulin sensitivity in the blood. When this happens, the body is at the optimum capacity to burn fat. Another helpful aspect for diabetes patients is that intermittent fasting also helps to reduce resistance to insulin. In the process, it lowers the blood sugar levels and also an individual's risk for type 2 diabetes.

Intermittent fasting can also increase the volume of **Human Growth Hormone (HGH)** naturally present in the bloodstream. When there are higher levels of Human

Growth Hormone in the body, an individual can burn fat while also gaining muscle.

This weight loss centers around an individual's belly fat, but still affects all fats deposited in the body. As your body is able to burn fat, it creates energy that continues a healthy cycle of healthy wellbeing.

At the cellular level, intermittent fasting can jumpstart one's cellular repair processes, including the removal of harmful wastes from the cells. The effects also show in reduced inflammation and oxidative stress and damage. The process of cleaning the blood system is known as **autophagy**.

During the repair process, the cells break down and metabolize proteins that have been deteriorating within the cells. When the body can properly go through the autophagy process, you will lower your chances of Alzheimer's disease and cancer.

Because your blood is being filtered through intermittent fasting, you will start to see improvement in your blood pressure levels, triglycerides present in the blood, and your total LDL cholesterol levels. The growth of new nerve cells will also protect you from damage to your brain.

Life Benefits of Intermittent Fasting

Your Day Will Be Simpler

You will not have to devote so much of your energy and time towards food preparation and shopping. There will be less stress in your life because you will have a set protocol to follow for the time to eat and then to fast. It takes a lot off your mind when you are not trying to find something to eat in a frantic stupor when the hunger pains strike.

You will also end up buying less food, which means you will spend less time shopping and you can devote that time to other activities.

Boost in Energy

Although you may run into some issues to start — as we all do when we try out a new lifestyle — you will notice that you suddenly have much more than you used to. You will have more energy to devote to other aspects of life that do not center around food.

If you are not thinking about food, you have more room to think about other important matters. Because your body is burning fat, you will also be lighter when you experience the energy boosts, telltale signs that you are becoming healthier.

Your Lifespan is Extended

Various studies have concluded that in rats, following the intermittent fasting lifestyle can extend life expectancy upwards to 83%. These findings are outstanding, and outline a major benefit to following intermittent fasting[28]. When coupling calorie restriction with fasting, it can increase an individual's overall lifespan.

During the process, aging is also slowed down, also helping to increase an individual's lifespan.

Easier Than Other Diets

Because you do not require a specific list of foods you need to eat, you can have fewer restrictions with this lifestyle. Intermittent fasting will also save you from searching for or buying specialized cookbooks and having to learn new recipes. As it was stated previously, following intermittent fasting will also help you with compartmentalizing your day.

Intermittent fasting makes your day easier to plan, and there are fewer interruptions.

You Will Save Time and Money

Because you will not be purchasing as much food, you will save money. In fact, you can save more if you find items on sale and freeze them or store them in the pantry for future meals when you are not fasting. Preparing double recipes and heating them up over the following few days is another great strategy.

When you do not spend as much time preparing meals throughout the day, **you save much valuable time.**

Chapter Summary

- Intermittent fasting is done over a specified amount of time where you abstain from solid food. You can still have calorie-free drinks during the fasting period.
- One of the main reasons people start with intermittent fasting is because it aids with weight loss. This is because the body becomes a fat-burning machine by using the stored sugars it saved up in the liver during fasting periods.
- Intermittent fasting simplifies your day because its schedule does not waste your time with food

preparation; it gives you a set schedule to follow to avoid unpredictability.

In the next chapter, you will learn about the myths associated with intermittent fasting.

Chapter 3: The Myths of Intermittent Fasting

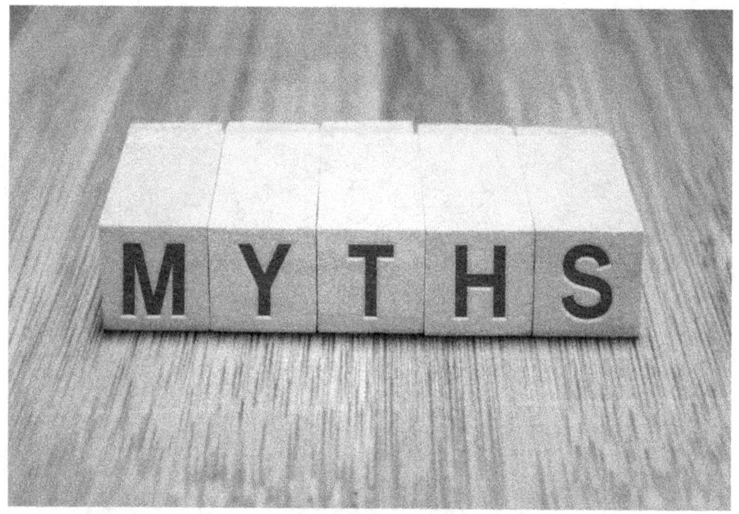

People associate intermittent fasting with several myths, despite how they all have no grounds whatsoever. The first of these myths that we are going to go over is that ***skipping breakfast makes you gain weight***. Many believe that breakfast is the most important meal of the day, and if you skip this meal, you will experience higher levels of weight gain, cravings, and hunger.

However, according to a study conducted on 283 adults over the course of 16 weeks, those who already suffer from obesity and weight issues saw no difference in their weight when they ate or skipped breakfast[6].

This study opposes the belief that one must eat breakfast to beat all weight issues. Although we cannot generalize to all individuals, this study still shows evidence that we may not necessarily need breakfast. There are those who have seen positive weight loss when they ate breakfast for a long-term duration[24]. The bottom line is that you need to listen to your body for what works for you personally.

A second major myth is that ***metabolism levels increase when you eat frequently***. Every time you eat, your body burns calories while your meals digest. This process is called the **thermic effect of food**, or **TEF**. When your body breaks down your food, it expands approximately 10% of the calories that you have just consumed on average. The problem with this concept is that people confuse how many times they eat compared to the number of calories burned.

For example, if you break up your meals into five meals throughout the day consisting of 400 calories, you will still consume about 2000 calories per day. However, using the 10% rule, you would only burn 200 calories for your digestive needs, which is the same amount of calories as if you were to eat only three meals a day. So as a result, eating more meals throughout the day does not allow you to eat more calories as the number of calories being used, regardless.

The next myth to address is the belief that you **reduce your hunger levels when you eat frequent meals**. This is a mixed truth myth, as the evidence to support or disregard the theory is also mixed. Some people swear by this belief, and it may actually work for them. Again, it comes down to listening to what your body is telling you; if it works for you to eat more frequently, then follow it, but if you find no difference, then you can follow your preference.

As far as evidence, there have been numerous studies that show there are no differences in hunger levels for those who ate more frequent meals versus those who did not[39, 42, 54, 55]. However, there was a study that concluded that when subjects consumed six high-protein meals divided throughout the day, they had fewer hunger pangs compared to those who ate three meals throughout the day[26]. This study shows that in some cases, frequent meals can reduce hunger levels.

In terms of frequent meals, another myth is that **splitting your meals throughout the day can help you lose weight**. Various studies have already proven that you cannot boost your metabolism solely by spacing your meals apart. However, there are other factors that may cause you to lose weight[16, 51].

In one study with 16 obese adults, there was no conclusive evidence that consuming smaller, more frequent meals throughout the day lead to any difference in their appetite or fat and weight loss[3].

Nevertheless, it helps some people stick to their diet goals when they can enjoy food throughout the day. Others are too tempted to overeat when given the opportunity to eat more frequently. If you find that you can succeed in splitting your meals, then you should incorporate frequent meals into your intermittent fasting plan.

Another common myth about intermittent fasting is that ***brain function will reduce if you do not consume dietary glucose regularly***. The idea is that you must consume soluble fiber approximately every three hours or the result will be that your brain will lose optimal functioning. This concept stems from the thought that your brain can only use glucose to fuel proper functioning.

However, your body is designed to produce glucose without introducing dietary fiber through a process known as **gluconeogenesis**. Your body can even produce ketones from fats present in the body when you are on a long-term fast. Your brain can then use these ketones as fuel. When this process occurs, you reduce the need to introduce glucose into the body, as your body requires little if no glucose to function.

Like with all diets, you should listen to your body. If you are experiencing symptoms of shaky body parts or fatigue, then you need to introduce the frequent eating system and perhaps keep some snacks handy throughout the day for convenience.

A common myth against intermittent fasting is that ***the periods of time you are fasting tricks your body that you are starving***. The idea is that when your body is in starvation mode, the processes of metabolism suspend, stopping the fat-burning process.

Studies have deduced that long-term weight loss plans can reduce the amount of calories burned during the day; however, this is the case for any followed weight loss plan[49]. As a positive, these studies also concluded that for the short-term, fasts can increase your metabolic rate. This result is from the extraordinary increase of norepinephrine within your blood. When this is present, it starts up your metabolism which results in body fat being broken down by fat cells[43, 66].

When metabolism was studied specifically, they found an increase between 3.6% and 14% when the fast was for a period of two full days. However, there is a balance to the fasting system because the longer you fast, the opposite effect takes place[30, 40, 66].

People also commonly believe that **you lose muscle mass when following the intermittent fasting diet**. It suggests that your body uses muscles for the fuel it needs during fasts. Overall, you will usually lose muscle mass while following any diet; however, there is no scientific evidence to support that intermittent fasting has a higher rate of muscle loss during the fasts.

In fact, there is evidence to support that you actually gain muscle mass through intermittent fasting. One study found that there was a minimal amount of reduction in muscle mass even with calorie restrictions[61]. This rings true for bodybuilders who use intermittent fasting for a lower percentage of body fat and also maintaining their required muscle mass.

The last of the myths we will cover here is the presumption that **following the intermittent fasting diet makes you consume more food**. There are some who believe that making yourself refrain from foods during extended periods will lead to eating more food during those eating windows. If an individual is not faithfully following the intermittent fasting diet, then consuming more food is entirely possible because the individual will feel like they need to compensate for the "lost" calories during the fast.

However, researchers have done studies on this subject and have found that participants who fasted for an entire day only consumed 500 calories the next day. This was a significant reduction in the 2,400-calorie diet that they were following before[23].

Another interesting study found that people who fast anywhere from three to 24 weeks could lose between four to seven percent of belly fat, and also between three to eight percent of their overall weight[1]. Overall, intermittent fasting has been proven through various studies that it will aid you in all your weight loss goals[10, 15, 16].

Chapter Summary

- One common belief is that weight gain will occur if skip "the most important meal of the day" — breakfast. However, this is not the case if have a healthy relationship with food.
- Another common myth that intermittent fasting will make you lose muscle mass because of the fasting process. Nevertheless, studies have actually found that it has the opposite effect.
- Some people believe that you must eat throughout the day so that hunger will not strike you. In this

case, you need to know the difference between physical hunger and psychological hunger.

In the next chapter, you will learn the differences between other common diets and intermittent fasting.

Chapter 4: Comparison of Intermittent Fasting with Other Diets

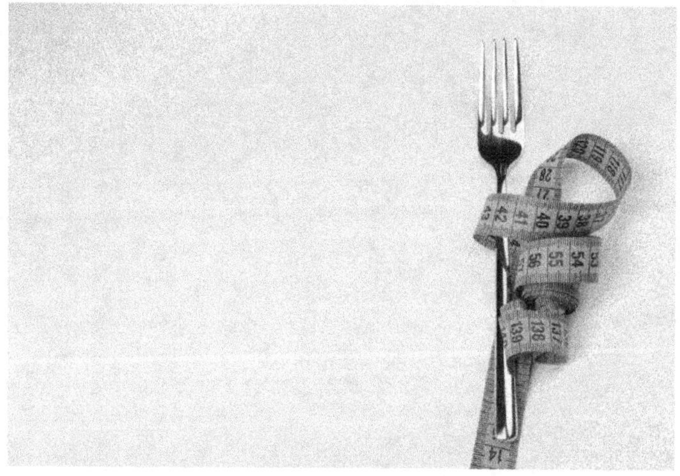

Not all diets are created equal. That is why there is such a wide variety of diets for all kinds of people. Here is an overview of the many popular diets out there today.

3-day Military Diet

This a low-calorie diet done over three days, where the individual eats anywhere from 1,100 to 1,400 calories. They can then return to regular eating on the 4th day. The diet is high in protein while low in calories, carbohydrates, and fat. It is designed to help people lose large amounts of weight in a short time by boosting metabolism to reduce amounts of fat in the body. People can lose up to a pound a day when following this regimen for a full month. However, the weight loss is over a short period before the user gains it back.

Keto Diet

This is a low-carbohydrate diet that eliminates foods with sugars and carbs to activate the fat-burning process. It is a diet that some people with gluten sensitivities usually decide to follow, coming out with positive results. There are a set amount of fat which the individual needs to consume and, and they need to keep carbs to six grams or fewer.

Similar to intermittent fasting, this is also a diet based on weight loss, but many of the same benefits appear in both.

Paleo Diet

This diet is considered non-traditional and focuses on eliminating processed foods. The diet consists of whole foods which include oils, fats, vegetables, fruits, nuts, seeds, eggs, fish, and meat. They also need to avoid eating artificial sweeteners, legumes, dairy products, and grains. The idea is to eat similar foods to what our ancestors ate thousands of years ago, as the food was much more natural.

Vegan

Veganism is not just a diet but an entire lifestyle. Because Vegans do not believe in harming animals, they refrain from eating any animals or bi-products, which would include any food item that was made with some animal involvement. This rule also extends to not wearing anything produced from different animal parts such as animal skins. Vegans also do not believe in supporting animals used for entertainment, or using any products tested on animals. Instead of consuming meat, they have a diet centered on whole grains, omega-3 fatty acids, vegetables, fruits, and nuts. Most vegans who choose this diet usually base their decision on personal preference rather than for any specific health reasons.

Intermittent fasting incorporates points from all these diets. Intermittent fasting allows for freedom to experiment with any of these diets too if you think they will personally help you eat healthier. You will need to be careful, however, as some of these diets are much more dangerous than others.

The most important aspect when looking to adopt a new relationship with food is to listen to what your body requires. You may find along the way that intermittent fasting methods simply do not work for your needs and current lifestyle. Despite this possible setback, you should never give up hope for achieving your goals because there will always be a way if you are determined enough.

Chapter Summary

- There are a surplus of diets that you can follow. One of them is the Keto Diet, where you cut out carbohydrates from your diet along with sugars and processed foods. Many people combine the Keto diet with Intermittent Fasting.
- The Paleo diet is a style of eating based on our ancestors' way of life; if it's not naturally produced, they do not include it in their diet.

- Vegans go one step further than those of the Paleo diet — they eliminate their entire consumption of animals and animal bi-products from their lives. This choice is more for personal reasons because they are distressed by the way society treats animals in general.

In the next chapter, you will learn about calories during intermittent fasting and ways that you can calculate your daily caloric intake.

Chapter 5: What are Calories and How to Calculate your Daily Intake?

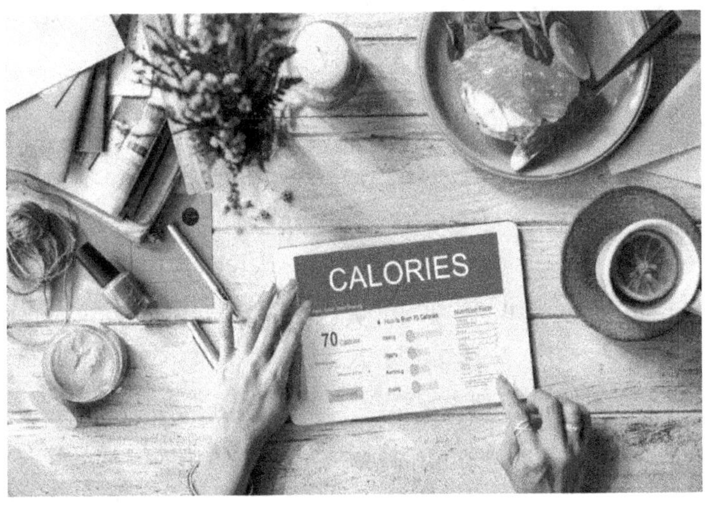

Calories give our bodies energy and are stored in body fat. Any time you read a nutrition label, you will see calories at the top of the list.. One calorie is divided into 1,000 kilojoules — what you read on nutrition labels is the broken down version of calories. 1000 kilojoules can be referred to as food calories, nutritional calories, dietary calories, or large calories. There are macronutrients which have a standardized amount of calories, and one gram of fat contains nine calories, whereas carbohydrates and proteins both contain four calories.

How Many Calories?

So how many calories should you consume in a day? This wholly depends on the resting metabolic rate of the individual and their activity levels. The average person will burn about 1,400 calories throughout the course of their day, which includes activities such as breathing, organ and digestive functions, and moderate exercise. As a baseline, women should not consume less than 1,200 calories, whereas men should consume a minimum of 1,500 calories; however, considering that this is just a baseline, it should be noted that everyone should consume different amounts of calories depending on their body type and level of exercise as well. The baseline calorie intake helps ensure that there is a healthy balance of micronutrients and major nutrients in the individual.

As stated, the basic guidelines created by health organizations dictate that one should consume a 2,000-calorie diet daily if they are female and upwards to 2,600 calories a day if they are male. Of course, it is possible to eat this amount of calories with just junk foods. According to the Dietary Reference Intake, you will want to consume between 45 and 65 percent of your calories from carbohydrates, between 20 and 25 percent from fat, and the remaining amount should be from proteins. These amounts are calculated for adults, as children require a higher amount of fat ranging from 25 to 40 percent of their calories.

When you are first starting out, you should track the amount of calories you eat. Not only with this help you keep on track with consuming a healthy amount of calories during your eating window, but you will also know if you are eating too much for your personal weight loss goals. When you can see the correlations between specific foods making you more energized or more irritable throughout the day, you will better know how to customize your eating plan to suit your body.

The **5:2 plan** is known to have an extremely low calorie count: between 500 to 600 calories on your eating days. You may find that you will need to eat more depending on how you feel, and especially when you first start with this method.

Calorie Calculators and Apps

The best way to figure out your daily calories is to use one of the calculators below to figure out how many calories you would typically burn in a day; this amount will still probably be around the 2,000-calorie mark. You can also take a different approach and eat a balanced diet until you are satisfied at each meal. Over time, this will work to lower your calorie count and you will start to see some weight loss.

Some people do not have the time to count the calories they are consuming. However, the following are helpful tools that will help you keep on track and can use easily and quickly on a tight schedule:

Calculator.net — This calculator will assist you in determining the amount of calories you need to consume during the day while also factoring in your level of fitness. It gives some guidelines for when you need to lose weight.

FreeDieting.com — This website tool gives you the amount of caloric intake you should focus on and can calculate the amount in pounds or kilograms. It also includes excellent weight loss tips.

Bodybuilding.com — Using this calculator, you can factor in the macronutrients you need to consume daily along with the intake of calories required for your fitness level and personal goals.

Studies have shown that people who use a log with record their calories are more prone to keep the weight off for a longer time[2, 22]. There are also several apps which are available which will help you calculate the calories you have eaten and burned. The best apps to assist in your weight loss are:

My Fitness Pal

This is the most popular app for anyone who wants to count calories. It records your weight and gives you the amount of calories you should eat every day, and can also tell you how many more calories you have to consume during your eating window. You may also use the included exercise log. This app is easy to use and has a webpage that syncs all your information.

You can set personal weight loss goals into the app and explore chat forums that can help to guide and support you. The chat includes personal success stories, tips, recipes, and conversions. There are thousands of recipes you can choose to download and save from the app for future reference.

The app also includes a pie chart that breaks down your fat, protein, and carbohydrate intake, along with a log for any notes you may have.

This app has a free download which allows you to access a limited amount of features. If you wish to upgrade to the premium version, it is at a cost of $49.99 annually. The app is available on iOS and Android, with a website as well.

Lose It!

This is also another popular health tracker that will follow your calorie count and log your exercise. You can also connect your fitness devices and pedometer to the app. On the homepage, you can track your calorie intake and calculate how many calories you should consume daily.

The program allows you to look up foods for their nutritional value, using helpful icons that show the food you are looking up. You can even use the app at the grocery store by scanning the barcode so you can store the food you buy for a more efficient process.

Included is a community chat that helps support all its members, and you can participate in daily and weekly goals. The app is free to download on both iOS and

Android devices. There is also a premium upgrade at the cost of $39.99 per year. With the upgrade, you can set more goals, view all of your statistics, and log additional notes for yourself.

FatSecret

This is a free app that can track your calorie intake, weight, and exercise, and allows for journal entries. It also includes a barcode scanner for easy entry of the foods you eat. On the homepage, it shows your total calorie intake and breaks down your fat, protein, and carbohydrates for each meal and throughout the day.

There is a monthly statistical view which compounds your information into daily and average totals. They also have a community chat with support, helpful tips, and recipes. Unlike the previous programs we have looked over so far, this app is completely free and is available for both iOS and Android. You also have the choice to use the website.

Cron-O-Meter

This handy app also lets you track your body weight and exercises. They even allow you to customize your account with specific diets such as vegetarian, low-carb, and the Paleo diet. In doing this, it automatically converts the amount of macronutrients and calories you should focus on each day.

They also have a food diary with a bar chart that breaks down your protein, fat, and carbohydrates daily with the calories burned. It also lets you know which vitamins and minerals you are receiving from all the food you consume.

The initial download is free to Apple and Samsung devices. They offer an upgrade for less than $3 per month which takes away the ads and also offers a more advanced analysis of your statistics.

SparkPeople

This is a fast growing application that features goals and progress, nutrition facts, and a calorie counter. It is easy to use, and you can input foods into your journal over several days if you ate the same thing each day.

There is a pie chart that breaks down your macronutrient levels of protein, fats, and carbohydrates, giving you the capability to customize your view.

The app also has a barcode scanner, so you can add in foods and recipes for quick results. There is an online community full of articles from wellness and health experts, recipes, and health news.

With the free version available on iOS and Android, you will be able to access one of the biggest online nutrition and food databases. However, you will need to upgrade to avoid ads and use more features ($4.99 per month, or $29.99 as a one time payment).

Chapter Summary

- Calories are in all the foods we consume, and they convert to energy within the body. A typical balanced diet will be an average of 2,000 calories daily.
- You will naturally consume a smaller amount of calories the longer you stick to intermittent fasting methods.
- Several calculators exist as apps and websites to help you figure out how many calories you need to consume to reach your weight loss goals. Other people may eat until satisfaction and learn naturally to consume fewer calories.

In the next chapter, you will learn about the different specific methods used in intermittent fasting. You can then determine which method will work best with your lifestyle.

Chapter 6: Techniques of Intermittent Fasting

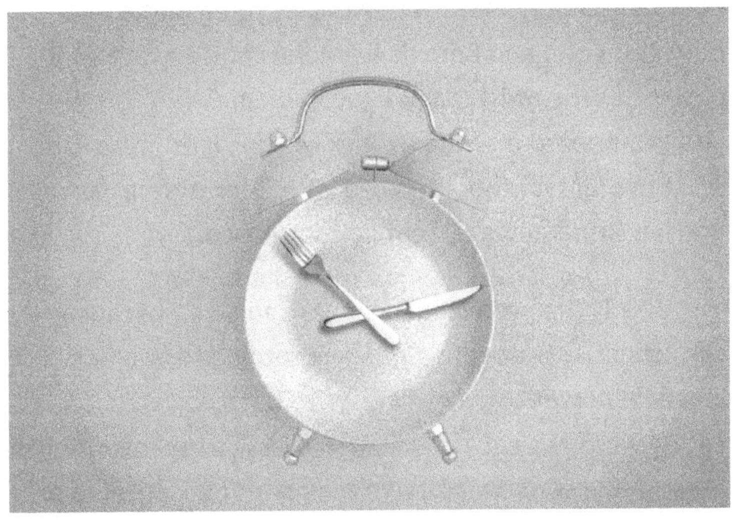

There are several intermittent fasting methods; they are what make intermittent fasting so easy to use because you can choose which method works best for your lifestyle. Here is a brief overview of the methods split into beginner, intermediate, and advanced fasting methods below:

Beginner Fasting

16:8 Pattern

Using this method, you would start by skipping breakfast each day and have a set eating window of eight hours; this could mean for example, you would eat between noon and 8pm daily. Many consider the 16:8 pattern as the most maintainable and most straightforward method to stick to. This method is the most popular method to begin with intermittent fasting, and it is also known as **Leangains Protocol**.

This is the preferred beginner's method because you can schedule your eating times according to your lifestyle; however, you will want to keep consistent eating windows each day. It is also easy to split your eight hour eating window into two meals, and it is ideal to do fasting exercise right before you break for your eating window. This meal should be your largest meal of the day, to refuel your body at your workout and fasting period.

When starting this fasting method, veteran fasters advise women to build up to the 16-hour fast by starting with 12 hours on the first day, then adding an hour each day until you have the full 16 hours of fasting.

5:2 Pattern

This method has you eating between 500 and 600 calories on two given days during the week and eating normally for the rest. These two days should *not be consecutive*. This pattern also goes by the name of the **Fast Diet**. During the two days of fasting, you cut back 75% of your normal food intake.

4:3 Pattern

This is plan involves eating 500 to 600 calories per day for three days of the week which can work out to every other day. You can drink water during your reduced-calorie fast. During the other four days of the week, you can eat a balanced diet as you would.

6:1 Pattern

This is a method for people who have been doing intermittent fasting for at least a month. You fast for one full day while you eat on the other 6 days of the week.

This can become more of a maintenance fast once you reach your ideal weight.

Alternate Day Fasting

Alternate Day Fasting (**ADF**) is as it sounds — you will eat as you would for one day. Then on the next day, you will fast completely for the full day; you may also have a 500 to 600 calorie diet on your fasting day to restrict your caloric intake. There have been positive results for heart patients who have followed this intermittent fasting method for the duration of six months. Users consume about 37% fewer calories per week while on this plan.

Eat-Stop-Eat Method

Also known as the **24-Hour Fast**, you would have a full day fast once or twice a week; you do not want to have these fasts back-to-back at any point during the week. You can do this as many days of the week as you wish; however, the normal amount you should do is to alternate days, which would work out to three times a week. This can begin at any point of the day that is comfortable for you. You can drink non-caloric fluids during this time. Once your fast is complete, you can eat again. With this method, you would consume at least ten percent fewer calories during a week period.

Warrior Diet

This is a 20-hour fast with a four-hour eating window. However, you may have some raw vegetables, fruits, and lean protein along with water during your fasting period. Setting the eating window to the evening and eating your meal in a specific order is ideal. You would start with the vegetables and fruit, then fats and proteins. You would then finish with carbohydrates if you are still hungry.

Periodic Fast

This is a 24-hour fast that does not use any eating or fasting schedule. You can try this when you know you will eat a heavy meal, such as a Thanksgiving or Christmas dinner. You can also do it when you will go on a long car ride so you may pass the time without thinking about food. This is an option for people with diabetes, as it lowers risk for any high or low blood sugar worries.

Intermediate Fasting

36 Hours

This is where you would only drink water and non-caloric drinks for 36 hours, and then you would have a 12-hour eating window. This is an effective way of eating 1,900 fewer calories during a week period.

48 hours

This is the longest fasting period traditionally practiced with intermittent fasting, with the two days of fasting are back-to-back. The best way to start this method is to begin the fasting period after dinner on the first day — you can then eat a sensible snack on the evening of the third day. About one to two hours later, you can have a small, balanced meal. You can drink non-caloric drinks and water during the two-day fast; it is important to stay hydrated during this form of fasting because dehydration is the true risk with longer fasting periods. You will only want to do this method once or twice a month, leaving about two weeks in between.

7 Days

People usually do this fast for spiritual purposes. It may be hard but it can have some fantastic health benefits. Not only will you clean out your system or any toxins you may have by drinking water and other non-caloric drinks, but you can even improve any medical symptoms you may have. It can also jumpstart your weight loss, but do not expect it to be a long-term change as the pounds will probably creep back in after you eat again. Gaining a better relationship with your food and making smarter food choices can help.

14 Days

The highly devout, such as monks or *babas* in the East, practice this form of fasting. If you are looking for a complete improvement to your health, bad eating habits, or food addictions, this option will help. You may drink water and drinks with no calories, but you would eat or drink nothing else while using this fasting practice.

When you follow one of these methods for an extended amount of time, you will reduce your overall calorie intake as long as you do not cheat by compensating during your eating window and consuming the lost calories during your fast[1, 19].

Chapter Summary

- There are several methods of fasting which you can use with intermittent fasting. The most common are the **16:8 Pattern** and the **5:2 Pattern**.
- These fasting methods allow you to drink water and other non-caloric drinks; this will aid your body in staying hydrated and also flush out any toxins present in your body.
- It is best to pick a method that will match your lifestyle best, but you want to be sure you can stick with your choice for at least three weeks before switching, unless you are using a method designed to only be used at irregular intervals.

In the next chapter, you will learn about the people who should exercise caution while performing intermittent fasting, and also how to tell if intermittent fasting is not right for you.

Chapter 7: Who Can Do Intermittent Fasting and What Precautions Should You Take?

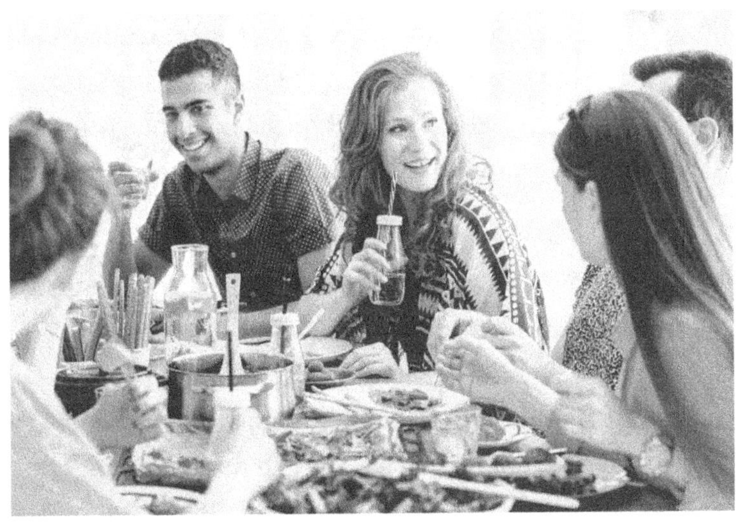

Unfortunately, medical professionals do not recommend intermittent fasting for everyone. Those who should refrain from following any intermittent fasting methods are those with a history of eating disorders or those who are already underweight. If fall into any of these categories, consult with your health professional before deciding to start intermittent fasting methods.

Certain studies have concluded that intermittent fasting *may not be as beneficial for women compared to men*[12]. Findings have seen insulin sensitivity improvements in men, but that blood sugar levels worsen in women.

Even though there has been no extensive research done on the benefits for men versus women, studies have found in rat studies that the female rats suffered from missed menstrual cycles, infertility and heightened masculinity while undergoing intermittent fasting methods[31, 32].

This case has also been true according to various personal stories of women who had missed menstrual cycles; these women also found that their menstrual cycles returned to normal after stopping their practice of intermittent fasting. If you experience missed periods while going through the intermittent fasting methods, stop fasting or try a more gentle approach. Likewise, if you are pregnant or breastfeeding, hold off on intermittent fasting.

For those with the following medical issues, consult with your medical doctor before considering starting with intermittent fasting methods:

- Female with a history of amenorrhea
- Female and trying to conceive
- Taking medications
- Low blood pressure
- Issues with blood sugar regulation
- Diabetes

Even if you fit any of these conditions, it does not mean that you cannot incorporate intermittent fasting in your life; however, there are precautions that your health professional will need to monitor.

When you are just getting started, follow the **16/8 method**. This form of fasting is the easiest to implement and you have likely already practiced this form of fasting before. This method would be when you sleep in one morning and your first meal that day is at lunch time. Once you are comfortable with this method, you can advance to the other methods such as **Eat-Stop-Eat** or the **5:2 method**.

Alternatively, you can test out your fasting capabilities by skipping a meal when you do not have the time to cook something proper or you are not hungry. This method is a great way to learn about listening to your body and its natural cycles, while also implementing some fasting techniques. When you start out, you will need to keep it simple. You will still see results from these first steps into intermittent fasting, no matter how small your lifestyle changes are.

One of the easiest ways to start is by cutting out all the unhealthy foods from your diet, including processed foods, sugar, and white bread. If it helps, try to eliminate one item each week to ease into the process. You also need to keep the meals you prepare as simple as you can. If you add in too many ingredients, you will also add more calories to the dish. Another tip is to switch the oil you use to non-vegetable oil, such as avocado oil or olive oil. Do not use margarine; substitute it with ghee and use *sparingly*.

Even if you find that intermittent fasting is not for you, this should not stop you from making healthier choices in the foods you consume. You can still go through all these steps and see changes in your weight and overall health. Never give up hope. You can try eating the Paleo or Keto diet for a while before you make it over the medical hurdles keeping you from using intermittent fasting methods.

Chapter Summary

- If you are pregnant, breastfeeding, have or have had a history with eating disorders, you should not follow an intermittent fasting plan, as it could damage your health.
- For those who have diabetes and heart disease, you will need to work with your health professional when undergoing intermittent fasting methods. They will monitor your health and adjust your medications as required.
- You can always make better choices in the foods you eat without going on a diet. Cut out one unhealthy food a week and you will notice how much more energy you have, and the weight will improve if you continue with this process.

In the next chapter, you will learn about the recommended foods and foods you will benefit the most from when coupled with intermittent fasting. You will also learn about the foods that you should avoid so you can reach ketones during your fasting period.

Part Two: Dos and Don'ts of Intermittent Fasting

Chapter 1: Intermittent Fasting Food List

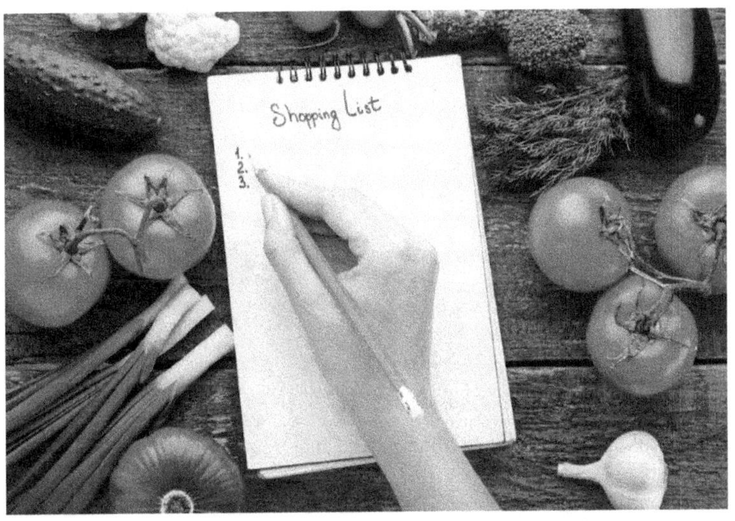

Even though there are no official foods list for intermittent fasting, there are a few guidelines which will make you more successful with your weight goals. You will want to refrain from certain high-fatty foods if you want to lose weight and refrain from eating high-calorie foods in the form of sweets and simple carbohydrates. These foods are the heavy hitters that will counteract your fasting process. The best way to succeed with intermittent fasting is to have a diet centered of lean proteins, dairy, seeds, beans, nuts, whole grains, veggies, and fruits. These foods are unprocessed, nutrient-dense, whole foods that are high in fiber.

Foods to Keep in Your Diet

- Water
- Fish
- Cruciferous Veggies
- Potatoes
- Beans and Legumes
- Probiotics
- Berries
- Eggs
- Nuts
- Whole Grains
- Coffee
- Red Wine
- Papaya
- Ghee
- Multivitamins
- Herbal Tea

- Olive Oil
- Coconut oil
- Yogurt
- Cream
- Lamb
- Seafood
- Nut Butters
- Chicken
- Cheese
- Seeds

Water

You need to keep yourself hydrated while fasting, especially during the fasting period. About 70% of your body is water, making it a vital component to ensuring your organs are working at optimum levels. If you are not keen on drinking water, you can add some flavor with lemon, lime, slices of cucumber, or a few mint leaves.

There are varied amounts of water everyone should consume, and the best way of knowing your hydration level is to look at your urine. The perfect shade is pale yellow, but if it is a darker shade, then this may indicate dehydration. Common signs of dehydrations are lightheadedness, fatigue, and headaches. These symptoms may become even more potent when you are not drinking enough water while also limiting your food intake.

You will find that you require more water when following intermittent fasting methods. While fasting, your body will search for energy pockets in your liver in the form of stored sugars known as **glycogen**. As the body uses this energy, it drains an immense amount of electrolytes and fluids. When you hydrate, you promote higher cognition levels, better blood flow, and also stronger joint and muscle support.

Fish

This food is an excellent source of protein and healthy fats. An added benefit is also the high amounts of Vitamin D. Fish is fantastic for brain function because of the omega-3 fatty acids, **DHA** and **EPA**. Keeping fish in your diet will help you deal with any brain fog you may experience while practicing intermittent fasting.

Cruciferous Veggies

These are foods such as cauliflower, Brussels sprouts, and broccoli, and are excellent for their high fiber content. When you are breaking up your eating habits, it is vital that you include fiber-rich foods. Not only will they keep your digestive tract in order, they will also keep you feeling fuller for longer.

Potatoes

Potatoes are perfect when combined with a protein source as a post-workout snack.

People can digest potatoes with little effort, and it will still refuel the muscles. They are also filling. Once cooled, they will form a resistant starch, excellent for feeding good bacteria present in your digestive tract; however, know that potato chips and French fries do not count.

Beans and Legumes

These foods are full of carbohydrates for supplying energy levels and are also low in calories with lots of fiber.

Foods such as lentils, peas, black beans, and chickpeas all fall into this category. Lentils will pull in 32 percent of your daily fiber intake with a half cup serving.

Beans and legumes are a definitive additive to women are following intermittent fasting too, as they are also good sources of iron — helpful to keep menses in check.

Probiotics

When you are experiencing symptoms of constipation, you may suffer from a bacteria imbalance, in which there are both healthy and damaging bacteria in your digestive system.

To help counteract this problem, you can consume kraut, kombucha, and kefir, which are all probiotic-rich foods. You can also use probiotic "shots" of juice which only have 10 calories per 1.5 ounces.

Berries

Smoothies are the best option during intermittent fasting. You can choose your favorite type of berry, but strawberries, raspberries, and blueberries are the optimum decisions because they carry essential vitamins keep you from erratic rising BMI levels. Blueberries contain high amounts of antioxidants, which will help you look younger and also increase your lifespan.

Antioxidants are ideal because they clean the body of free radicals and protect your cells from damage.

Eggs

Eggs are an excellent source of protein and are easy to cook up in less than five minutes. Another added benefit is that they are also filling. When you add eggs to your diet, you consume sufficient amounts of protein and your muscles will build. Eggs are also a diverse food, which means there are many ways to prepare it. Two whole eggs a day guarantee a good intake of choline and vitamins. Eggs improve the physical performance of athletes. The nutritional value of egg is better when the yolk is still liquid after cooking.

Nuts

Although nuts can be rather high in calories, they are an excellent source of polyunsaturated fat, meaning they can make you less hungry and satiated longer. If you worry about calories, studies have found that almonds have about 20 percent fewer calories than listed on the packaging. Almonds have fewer calories is because chewing the nuts does not crush them entirely, leaving the unchewed portion to pass through your digestive system[41].

Other great benefits to consuming nuts include burning fats and lengthening your lifespan. There are also ongoing studies that suggest nuts can reduce your risk of early mortality, type 2 diabetes, and cardiovascular disease[23].

Whole Grains

Eating carbohydrates is not always welcome when you are trying to lose weight; however, whole grains are full of protein and fiber. Not only will they keep you full for longer, but you will also boost your metabolism. Some types of whole grains are freekeh, sorghum, millet, amaranth, kamut, spelt, bulgur, and farro. Indulging in whole grains means that you can enjoy sliced breads, crackers, and bagels while still following intermittent fasting.

Coffee

This calorie-free beverage is a favorite among the intermittent fasting crowd, and people practicing intermittent fasting can even consume it during fasting periods without a problem, but you *must* take it straight. Remember that while fasting, you cannot add any sugar, flavorings, or a large amount of cream or milk to the beverage.

Red Wine

Red wine has polyphenols from the grapes used in its making, which some studies have concluded cause red wine to have anti-aging effects. Fear not — you can enjoy a relaxing glass of wine every once in a while when using intermittent fasting methods.

Papaya

You will start experiencing hunger pains a few hours into your fast, and as a result, you may overeat during your eating window, causing fatigue and bloating. The beauty of adding papaya into your diet is that it contains an enzyme known as **papain**, which breaks down proteins. This breaking down of proteins means that when you enter back into your eating window, you will eat a protein-rich meal that will assist you with an easier digestion.

Ghee

When looking at the different oil options, most people know about the health benefits of olive oil; however, ghee is another healthy oil to consume. People overlook it, despite its benefits. People can use it while preparing hot dishes, as it has a high smoke-point.

Multivitamins

Not consuming the same amount of food you were before can raise the risks of having a vitamin deficiency. When you combine a healthy balance of vegetables and fruits into your diet, you can lower your chances for vitamin deficiency, but if you find that you are lacking in vitamins, a multivitamin can be a convenient way to receive the nutrients your body requires. If you can, take vitamins of natural origin rather than synthetic vitamins.

Herbal Tea

This drink is an excellent choice to have during your fasting periods and throughout intermittent fasting. Some good choices for herbal teas are spearmint, peppermint, ginger, red tea, and chamomile. Just like water, herbal teas will keep your body hydrated without putting a stop to your fat-burning process.

The change in flavors can also be refreshing.

Olive Oil

Olive oil, especially extra virgin olive oil, is an excellent ingredient for weight loss. It is full of monounsaturated fatty acids, which keeps your heart healthy, your blood sugar levels stable, and help assist weight loss. Indeed, by promoting the feeling of satiety, it prevents you from bingeing on other refined or trans-fat sources laden with empty calories. It is so much healthier than other fat sources like butter and refined oil. According to experts, it is much better than sesame, rapeseed, sunflower and corn oil!

Coconut Oil

This oil is high in saturated fats and has a higher heating point, meaning that you can use it in almost any meal that you make. It is an excellent fat burner because of the **medium-chain triglycerides (MCTs)**, which will also help you burn more calories[38].

Another study concluded that between fifteen to thirty grams of MCTs per day increases your energy levels, helping you to burn an additional 120 calories per day[56].

Seeds

Adding seeds to your diet will help you reduce blood pressure, blood sugar, and cholesterol. The best seeds to add to your intermittent fasting regimen will be flaxseeds, sunflower seeds, chia seeds, hemp, sesame seeds, and pumpkin seeds.

Yogurt

Yogurt is an excellent source of calcium and protein, and it also helps you balance out your digestive system. It relieves *irritable bowel syndrome* and protects your bones against *osteoporosis*. Make sure you purchase yogurt with no sugar added; Greek yogurt is a popular non-sugar yogurt choice. It can also be a great addition to your first meal once you finish with your fasting period.

Cheese

Cheese is a great source of protein, fat, and calcium. There is also a high content of vitamins and minerals such as A, B12, zinc, riboflavin, and phosphorus. These vitamins and minerals will help your body maintain receiving nutrients it craves after your fasting period.

Chicken

Chicken is one of the best choices you can make while practicing intermittent fasting. It is high in protein, meaning it is also low in fat. You can build up your muscle mass when you consume chicken and other lean meats.

Chicken is also high in niacin, vitamin B6, phosphorus, and selenium.

Lamb

Lamb is another type of lean meat high in protein. Several essential vitamins and minerals exist in lamb, including vitamin B12, zinc, and iron. It also aids in muscle growth, energy, and maintenance of the muscular system.

Seafood

Shrimp, lobster, salmon, tuna, and mackerel are all high in fats, meaning they will help to boost your system with the energy it needs during your long fasts.

Nut Butters

Nut butters are full of vitamins and minerals, even though people forget about them. Some, like coconut butter, are also antibacterial and will help you keep your health at optimum levels. Examples of nut butters include almond butter, coconut butter, hazelnut butter, and grass-fed butter.

Foods You Want to Avoid

- Processed Foods
- Sugar
- Caffeine
- Artificial Juice
- Sugary Fruits
- Root Vegetables
- White Carbohydrates

Processed Foods

These are foods loaded with preservatives so they can last longer on the shelves and in your freezer; the preservatives they add make processed foods not whole nor nutrient-dense like the foods you should consume. In fact, they are more full of fat and carbohydrates. Your body cannot process foods of this nature easily, putting a real strain on your system whenever you eat them.

Sugar

In today's society, sugar is an additive found in many foods, and especially in processed foods. This overload of sugar in the modern-day diet is not healthy and can lead to weight gain and other major health issues. It is important to consider that other sweeteners, such as honey or agave, can still pose health risks despite being slightly healthier choices. When you consume sugars, it causes a spike in your blood sugar which will then release insulin into the bloodstream, putting a stop to your fasting process.

Zero-calorie sweeteners, such as sucralose and stevia, can also trigger insulin production.

Caffeine

Many people consume caffeine for the boost in the energy it supplies; however, this state is temporary. Many foods and drinks, including green and black tea, contain some amount of caffeine. When you consume caffeine, it blocks the receptors for **adenosine**, the chemical that makes you sleepy. The "crash" you experience after is because the adenosine is merely *blocked*, not taken out — adenosine rushes out quickly and in high volume once the caffeine wears off, making you tired, and sometimes, irritable. Be careful when you consume coffee during your fasting period because combining no nutrients along with a caffeine crash can be detrimental. Some people can also experience heartburn, indigestion, mood swings, and physical jitters when consuming caffeine on an empty stomach.

Artificial Juice

These are juices made from concentrate to mimic the flavoring on the label. Other additives in these juices can help enrich the flavor, but they are not natural. Even though they may be more water than juice, this beverage is not a good option for intermittent fasting because of the added sugars included.

Sugary Fruits

These are tricky, as you can eat fruits during intermittent fasting. However, some fruits such as oranges, peaches, and plums are naturally high in sugars. Even though they are natural sugars, consuming these fruits will fill your liver with glucose, counteracting the effects of your fasting periods.

Root Vegetables

Root vegetables are high in starchy carbohydrates which will convert into sugar in your system and will counteract with your efforts during your fasting period. Some examples are carrots, sweet potatoes, turnips, beets, and radishes.

White Carbohydrates

Also known as **gluten**, this is the main product in white bread products. Often, people may have issues with digesting gluten and not realize gluten itself is the problem. You may try the Keto diet which, as explained, you can combine with intermittent fasting and cut out gluten altogether.

White carbohydrates will also wreak havoc with your glucose levels and make it difficult for your body to enter kinesis.

The Process of Ketosis

When you are confident that you can follow these food guidelines, your body will go into the state of **ketones** during your fasting periods. Ketosis is a medical expression that defines the state of the body when you produce ketones from fat consumption. Your body ordinarily produces glucose from carbohydrate intake,which is where the body receives its source of energy. However, if carbohydrate ingestion is too high, it can cause weight gain and health complications.

Ketones are an important chemical because it is the goal for your liver to create these ketones, which is the fat in your body being recycled for fuel. This process occurs when there is a deficit of insulin in your body. The insulin's responsibility is to transfer the glucose into the energy you need to function every day.

Most of the information studied about ketones is for people who have fasted because the process of ketones starting when the body spends the carbs present, making the liver create ketones to make up the deficit. When you fast for longer than 72 hours, the liver will create even more ketones.

There is a balance with how many macronutrients you should consume to keep the level of ketones you desire in your body on the Keto diet. If you, for example, eat too many proteins, your insulin levels will rise. As we learned, this will take your body out of ketones, resulting in the insulin creating sugars that your body is inclined to use for fuel and stops producing ketones in the liver.

Because you will ingest a lower amount of carbohydrates, your body will use the stored sugars and fats in your liver to help you eliminate the fat stored in your body. The result is the weight loss people work for when following intermittent fasting protocols.

Chapter Summary

- Even though much of the information on the internet says that you can eat whatever you want while following intermittent fasting, it is ideal to eat a balanced diet so you may benefit even more from the practice.
- There are many healthy foods on the list that you can eat, which will be full of nutrients that your body will crave after your fasting period is over.

- Even though you may think root vegetables are healthy, they can still spike your sugar levels and are best avoided.

In the next chapter, you will learn about planning out your meals and gain new ideas for meal preparation that will save you time and money. You will also be given some guidelines on what to eat and how to build up to your first 16-hour fasting period.

Chapter 2: Meal Planning for Intermittent Fasting

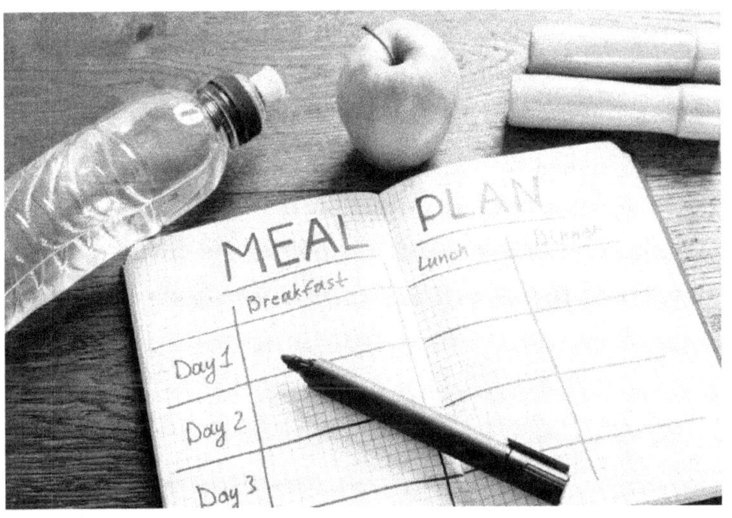

The Basics of Meal Prepping and Planning

There are many advantages to meal prepping and planning that you may not think about. The main benefits are that you will save a lot of time and also a lot of money, and we all know that we need more of both!

To plan out your meals ahead of time, you will need to create a shopping list. If you use a shopping list, you can stay within your budget by not buying unnecessary food that may go bad in your fridge before you can have them. It also gives you a chance to see what you have on hand, and you may learn that you need not go shopping at all.

When you go to the store, it will be best to avoid the aisles that will tempt you the most, such as the sweets aisle or the chips aisle. As a general rule, do not shop when you are hungry, as that will be another state in which you may end up buying more than you need. Avoiding certain aisles will also help keep you within your budget and to stay on track with your new lifestyle.

Because you will cook the meals ahead of time and bring your meals with you to the office or the gym, the snacks and meals you used to eat will no longer tempt you.

You can also double or triple the recipes you make to help keep you on course, and it will save you time from having to cook meals throughout the day.

Example of a Weekly 5:2 Plan

*Note: Do **not** schedule the **fasting days** back-to-back.*

Day 1

Breakfast: Poached Egg with whole wheat toast. One serving of grapes.

Lunch: Steak and mashed potatoes. Side of kale.

Dinner: Vegetable soup. One small salad drizzled with olive or coconut oil.

Day 2

Breakfast: Burrito made with small whole wheat tortilla wrap filled with two strips of grilled lean bacon, half an avocado, and one sliced tomato.

Lunch: Ham salad made with two tablespoons of potato salad, tomato, and green bell pepper.

Dinner: Pan-fried fish and asparagus, cherry tomatoes, couscous, and broccoli.

Day 3

Breakfast: Two scrambled eggs. Side of cherry tomatoes and mushrooms.

Lunch: Three whole wheat crackers and feta cheese. Top with cucumber, celery, and bell pepper.

Dinner: Whole wheat bun burger. Chicken patty with lettuce, tomato slices, raw red onion rings, and one teaspoon salsa. One apple.

Day 4

Breakfast: Tropical fruit salad with pineapple, bananas, and grapes. Mixed with Greek yogurt and one teaspoon of pine nuts.

Lunch: Open rye sandwich with lettuce, tomato, red onion slices, and three slices of cooked chicken.

Dinner: Six prawn kebabs; alternative could be tomatoes onto skewers. Brush with one teaspoon of olive oil. Side of a red onion and a green salad drizzled with olive oil.

Day 5

Breakfast: Blueberry smoothie with one small mango, three tablespoons Greek yogurt, and half a cup of low-fat milk.

Lunch: Tomato salad with chopped cucumber, chopped red onion, and green bell peppers. Garnish with basil leaves, minced garlic clove, and one teaspoon of olive oil.

Dinner: Tuna, mashed potatoes, and green beans.

Fasting Days

Drink water, herbal or fruit tea, and black coffee. Do not add sugar to any of the drinks, or you will pull your body out of fat-burning mode. Try to keep coffee to three cups maximum.

The first week is crucial for setting your intermittent fasting goals and to determine which method is right for you. You will want to ease into intermittent fasting so you do not shock your system or find it too difficult and quit shortly after starting.

When you choose your first method, you will want to continue for a duration of *three weeks* before you think about switching to another method.

You should split your eating windows into two meals with an optional snack, as it will ensure that your weight loss is effective during the entire process of intermittent fasting.

How to Build Up Fasting Hours

This is a **first five-day guide** for you if you are just starting with intermittent fasting. It might be tough at first, but this plan will guide you in how to build the hours of fasting that you perform. Once you complete the five days, you will have officially started the 16/8 Method.

Day 1 — 12-hour eating window & 12-hour fasting window

Day 2 — 11-hour eating window & 13-hour fasting window

Day 3 — 10-hour eating window & 14-hour fasting window

Day 4 — 9-hour eating window & 15-hour fasting window

Day 5 — 8-hour eating window & 16-hour fasting window

After this point, you will have worked yourself up to a 16-hour fasting window. Keep up the good work!

Chapter Summary

- It is important to plan out your meals for the week. This way you can shop once a week for the ingredients you require and make several meals at once to save some time.
- Make sure you consume enough calories each day while also ensuring that you will feel full afterwards so you will not be inclined to cheat during your fasting period.
- You can build up to a 16-hour fasting period by starting off at 12 hours on the first day and adding an hour each day for 5 days.

In the next chapter, you will learn about eating out at restaurants and how to not blow all your calories for the day on one meal.

Chapter 3: Tips for Dining Out with Intermittent Fasting

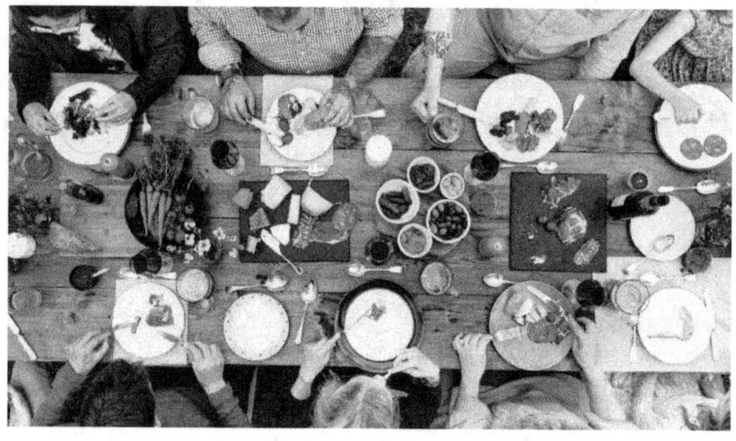

Just because you have made this choice to follow intermittent fasting to better your life does not mean you have to put your social life on hold — you just need to take a different approach. If someone or a group invites you out to dinner, *be sure* it is not during your fasting period. It will only tempt you because you will think you are being antisocial if you do not participate in eating a similar amount of food as everyone else.

You can do a little homework ahead of time if you plan to go to a new location. Search to see if they have an online menu that you can review ahead of time. Use an online menu to help you decide what you can eat before you arrive. Once you can decide on a meal, you will not be under the pressure of figuring out what you should eat while you are there, and you will not have to worry about going over your calorie count.

If the menu is not available online, try to give the restaurant a call to inquire if they have dishes you can enjoy while fasting. Perhaps they have a fruit or vegetable appetizer or plate that you can order. Inquire if they have whole-grain breads and any other particular foods you are abstaining from.

When you arrive at the restaurant, ensure that the item you had picked out is still available and review the menu to see if there are any changes. When you order your meal, make sure you know the item's ingredients, especially if they are using vegetable oil to prepare your meal, as you have a right to know. If you have an influence in terms of where you plan to go, you can also eat out at a restaurant you have been to before and of which you already know the menu. It is even better if you know how they prepare the food so you do not have to do your homework ahead of time.

Just because you are going out to celebrate or hang out with friends, does not mean that you have to go overboard on your meal. Celebrations and hangouts are not opportunities or excuses to eat terrible foods or overeat. You need to remember your "why" for what made you want to do intermittent fasting In the first place so you can keep your priorities straight. This way you will stay on track, while still enjoying yourself.

When you can fight the urges and discipline yourself accordingly to reach your goals, then it shows just how much you love yourself.

Chapter Summary

- Even though you may set yourself on a specific intermittent fasting method and schedule, it does not mean that you have to become a hermit; you can still have a social life. It is just going to be a little different.
- Be sure you study the menu before you arrive at a restaurant, or call to find out if they have a meal you can enjoy guilt-free.
- You can also go to a restaurant where you have been before and already know the ingredients and preparation of your favorite meal.

In the next chapter, you will learn about the common mistakes that people make while going through the process of intermittent fasting and how to counteract these mistakes so you do not fall into the same traps.

Chapter 4: Common Mistakes During Intermittent Fasting

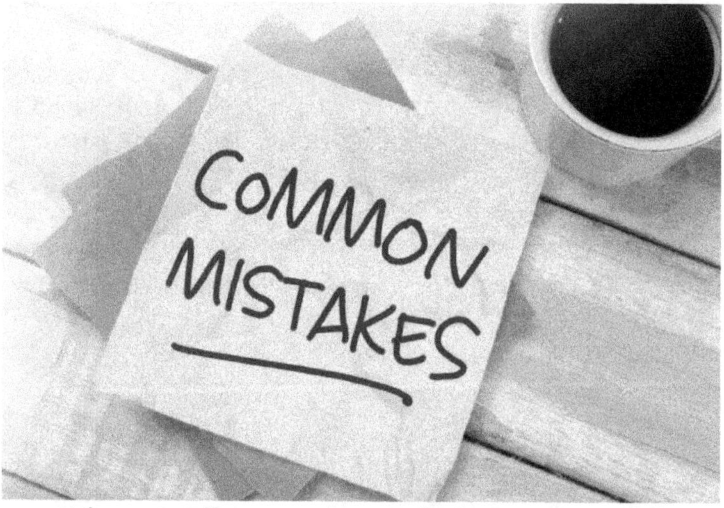

When you do not understand where you can fail, you will fall into specific habits without knowing it. However, when you educate yourself about the obstacles you will face, you will require less effort to overcome them, and you will also find success on the other side.

Eating Junk Food During Your Eating Period

Some people believe that intermittent fasting works like magic no matter what you eat. This is an insensible claim because becoming healthier cannot happen if the person is still eating sugar and processed foods. You must eat a balanced and nutrient-dense diet for intermittent fasting to be effective to its full capacity because your body breaks down the nutrients for energy during the fasting period. If you eat junk food, you will clog your system and feel terrible. Eating a whole-food diet will help you from feeling hungry during these fasting periods.

Not Eating Enough Calories During the Eating Window

It is common for those who have just begun with intermittent fasting methods to keep their calories to a minimum during their eating window. The thought behind this belief is that the fewer calories consumed, the more weight you will lose. You will instead need to split up your total count of calories between your two meals during your eating window. This strategy will help your body function at its optimal level so you can burn fat at a healthy pace.

Making Too Many Changes at One Time

This mistake can include under or overeating, training or exercising too hard, or starting with a long fast that your body has not prepared for. There is nothing wrong with entering intermittent fasting with an enthusiastic attitude toward making positive lifestyle changes; however, you need to listen to what your body is telling you during this process. If you change everything all at once, you will not know if it is working or if your method needs adjusting.

With any major lifestyle change, it is best to ease into the process. This way, you will give your body time to adjust to all the new changes. So, instead of training at the gym for five days a week after you have been running every once in a while, start with two or three times a week and build your tolerance levels up. Then incorporate the fasting schedule at a gradual pace. Try changing one thing per week until your body is ready and prepared.

Obsession with Eating and Fasting Windows

It is easy to think that you need to fast for a certain amount of hours at first. However, intermittent fasting should be on a trial-and-error basis. Until you can listen to your body and get more in tune with it, you will not know if your particular method works out for you, or if it does not.

At first, it is best to build this relationship between you and your body. Learn what signs your body shows when you are experiencing actual hunger instead of boredom, frustration, or habit. This is the chance for you to become in line with what your body requires. It is also a way to feel fuller during the fasting period.

Chapter Summary

- It is a common issue for people to overeat when they are just enter the eating window. Overeating will lead to digestive issues and a bloated feeling.
- Many people are eager to start the intermittent fasting program so they can see the changes it can bring. You may set yourself up for failure if you change everything at once, however.
- Do not stress yourself out so much about your eating windows and fasting times. The point is to become more in tune with your body and give it what it needs. Go with the process.

In the next chapter, you will learn how to stick to your original goals when you start intermittent fasting.

You will learn to keep your motivation and move towards your goals even when times are tough.

Chapter 5: Best Practices for Sticking with Intermittent Fasting

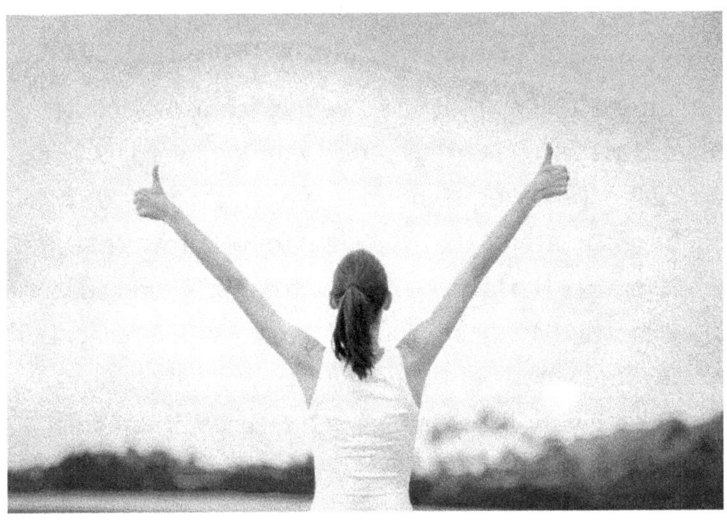

When you make your mind up to do something, you make a routine that ensures you complete it. When you do this plan over a certain period, about 28 days, it becomes a hard-to-break habit; this habit has become a part of who you are. You will want to make a routine and plan to rise above the challenges you will face when practicing intermittent fasting.

You may have a hard time drinking enough water, so you would then focus on drinking more water for the first week. If you have a problem with sugars, perhaps try to cut back your consumption by half. Not everything has to have a drastic change, as it is always better for you to do what is most comfortable for you personally because all of this work is for your own betterment.

Other ways that you can make sure you continue to build success with intermittent fasting is to find something healthy that you love to eat and use it as a **reward system**. We are wired to want a reward for a job well done; however, sometimes we tend to over do it. So, have something that you want to work toward, whether that is a favorite healthy treat or a trip you have been meaning to make. You need to have several goals to stay motivated because not every day will be easy. But if you keep your head up high and focused on the final prize, you will get there.

When you can set small goals and reach them with consistency, it will build your confidence in knowing that you can perform well with intermittent fasting. You will also be able to motivate yourself through the tougher days or through what may seem like a never ending fast. It can also help to have a project or activity that you have not had the time to do to keep your mind occupied during your last few fasting hours when your thoughts center around food again. Having that distraction will be healthier in the long run.

If have a hard time staying focused on your own, finding a friend on social media or in real life who can cheer you on through the process is a great idea. They need not participate in the intermittent fasting method, but someone supportive of you as a person will work great. This person should also be someone whom you have mutual respect and who will tell you how you can improve if you slip. They will be there for you through the thick and thin of the whole process and will cheer with you when you meet your personal goals.

If you are having problems in focusing on your *why* during the rough times, take a moment to sit down in a quiet place to calm your mind through meditation. It does not have to take a lot of time out of your day, and you can do it just about anywhere. Focus on your breath in how it is flowing in and out of you. You can focus your mind on your why and make it into a mantra, or you can try to free your mind from your racing thoughts. You do this by acknowledging a thought that comes into your head and letting it go; do not spend any time dwelling over that thought. Continue the process until you have no more racing thoughts.

If you are having a tough time getting through a particular fasting period or your body is feeling ill from the changes taking place, know that nothing is permanent. If you focus on the bigger picture than what seems like your problem in that very moment, you will find that it is all going to be worth it. Once you get past the rough patches, you will know what to do by keeping your mind on the overall prize.

Do not think you are a big shot and start an intermittent fasting routine that you cannot handle. It is okay to start from scratch and build yourself up, and it is also alright if you need to eat a restricted diet on your fasting days until you build up your strength. You need to be kind to yourself throughout the process, otherwise you will end up setting yourself up for failure for making your personal bar too high. Do not worry about anyone else but yourself and stay in the moment. Enjoy the process for everything that it is, as going through intermittent fasting will help you achieve your health goals.

If you find that intermittent fasting is just too difficult for you, it is okay to take a break from it for a day or two. This way, you can gather up your strength, courage, and determination once again to tackle your goals. Never do yourself the disservice of quitting because this is your life we are talking about. However, you need to look out for your overall health. If you think the method you are using is not right for you, stop and try something different. Nothing will keep you from realizing your goal if you want it badly enough.

Chapter Summary

- Once you start a new routine, over a period of about 28 days, it will become a habit. It will then become second nature and will be how you live your life from then on.
- Do not panic and give up in the middle of the process. There are millions of people who have gone through this same process, and there are people who made it through the same things you did. Never give up.
- Keep your mind calm and occupied. Be sure to have some projects you have been meaning to tackle in case your mind focuses on hunger or the time.

In the next chapter, you will learn about several apps that you can use to work towards your health goals.

Chapter 6: Apps to Keep you on Track in Intermittent Fasting

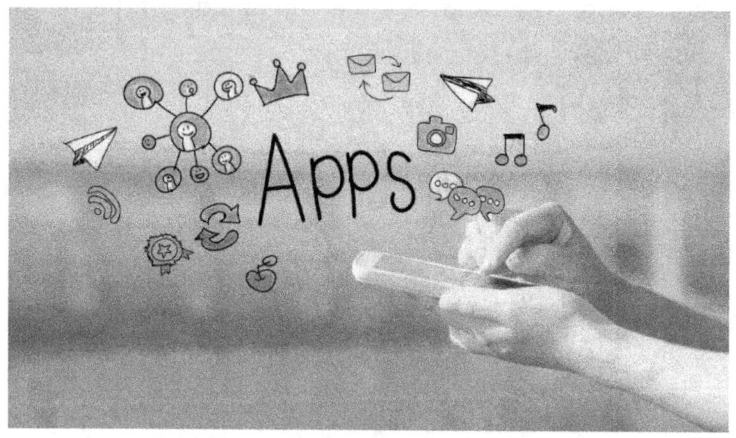

There are several apps out on the market which can help you stay on track with your goals.

They are all unique, so read on to find out which app will work best for your needs.

BodyFast

This app is the highest ranked in terms of its abilities and specificity for intermittent fasting, with over six million users. You can make a personal weight loss plan and download it on both iOS and Android phones. It comes in multiple languages, including Italian, French, Spanish, Portuguese, German, and English. You can have an individual coach included with the premium version who will calculate the best fasting plan based on your personal goals, and there are also weekly goals that you can complete which will continue to push you to strive towards improvement. The app, without the premium version, is free to download.

Overall, there are ten fasting plans on the app, and it works on a trophy system for when you achieve your goals. The premium version is just over $5 a month; even if you do not want to pay for an upgrade, you can still use the features of the app. The coach is also there to be your cheerleader and to guide you through your personal experience with intermittent fasting.

FastHabit

This app, available on iOS and Android, can keep a running log of your fasting periods. This easy-to-use app will also set up reminders for fasting periods and for eating windows. You will have many processes for following your progress and to see the statistics for the last ten days you have used the program. This app is free to download.

You can also input your fasting history manually, and they would track your streaks within the app. They have a premium version which is $2.99 per month, which adds the ability to see the last ten days of your fasting and look ahead at what is in store for your next ten days. You can also view more statistics and you will have more notifications and reminders compared to the regular version.

MyFast

This is another popular app with 200,000 users. You can plan out an eating schedule that you prefer, and you can use multiple devices with information shared between each. This app is entirely customizable, which gives you control over the notification settings, using metric or imperial units, time and date format, and language.

This app goes further because it allows you to record your weight and fasting windows while being able to export the information to a .CSV file; you will then be able to visualize your progress. There is also information included about intermittent fasting where you can find out the answers to questions you may have and also read about the benefits of intermittent fasting. You can download this app on iOS or Android systems for free.

Even though the ratings are lower for this app compared to the others, there are specifics which may help some users. First off, it keeps things all on the home screen with a button to begin a fast, the time since your last fast ended and your fasting goal length. It is a little more difficult to set up your personal goals as there are many screens before you get to the specific settings.

Track Your Fast

Whether you have been doing intermittent fasting for some time or are merely a beginner, you will find this an easy app to use. It also comes with a widget that can show your progress without the need to unlock your phone. There is a countdown for your fasting period and the ability to track your personal weight loss goals.

At the moment, this app is only available for Android devices. There is a premium version that you can purchase for $1.99 that will remove pop-up ads. The upgrade also allows you to view your weight loss progress.

<u>Vora</u>

This app has the same features as the other apps that we have covered; however, they go a little further. It has a real-time tracker which will guide you through the amount of weekly you have set to fast along with your actual numbers and a heat map. Vora is available on both iOS and Android, and they have a social platform for members to communicate and support each other. It is the number one app on Reddit for fasters. There is a required registration before you use the app, but you can monitor your progress after registration as everything is accessible through the main screen.

<u>Zero</u>

With this app, you can set your fasting periods up to a week ahead, and has an added feature with a notes section so you can record how you feel once you terminate your fast. You may also include anything else relevant that happened during your fast time in your notes. There are many sources of information about intermittent fasting available in the form of podcasts, videos, articles, and studies. You can pick fasting periods between 13 and 16 hours, or set up your own custom fasting schedule. You can also download your statistics to a .CSV file if you want to see information that is more than a week old. It is free for both iOS and Android.

Fastient

This is a well-rounded app found on iOS, Android, and online. It has comprehensive information and stats about your fasting times, calories burned, weight you have lost, a countdown for your fast, and an input for fasting time goals. It includes a journal where you can record any notes to yourself so you can write about your personal experiences during your intermittent fasting. You can also see your statistics on a monthly basis to track your progress with total weight loss and longest fasting time.

There is a registration required which will allow you to have all of your information synced together, whether you use your phone or web-based application. It is a free download, and there are no upgrades required to use all of its features. You can import a .CSV file of your previous fast times and weight stats so you can use the app even if you have been using others in the past. The app allows you to customize the time and date, and it also allows for the use of imperial and metric systems.

<u>Nightfast</u>

This is a newer app which is only available on Android products. It simple to use — just input your fasting window and you are ready to begin. You will get a notification for when your fast is complete and can view your fasting history, as the app saves it to your device. It is also possible to input past fasts into the app manually if you wish. There is also a way to track your weight loss and input a goal for a specific amount of weight loss.

The app does not contain a lot of clutter, which makes it easy to navigate. It contains other fasting plans including the intermittent fasting methods such as **circadian rhythm fasting** and the **One Meal a Day (OMAD)** diet. It is free to download, and there is no upgrade at the current time.

Chapter Summary

- Apps are the best way in today's society to keep in touch with your progress toward your goals.
- There are only two out of the list which you can only download on Android; however, the rest are available for you to download on any device.
- Often, an upgrade is necessary to enjoy the full range of a fasting app. However, the costs are reasonable, and contain many benefits.

In the next chapter, you will learn about the commonly asked questions about intermittent fasting and the honest answers.

Chapter 7: Common Frequently Asked Questions About Intermittent Fasting

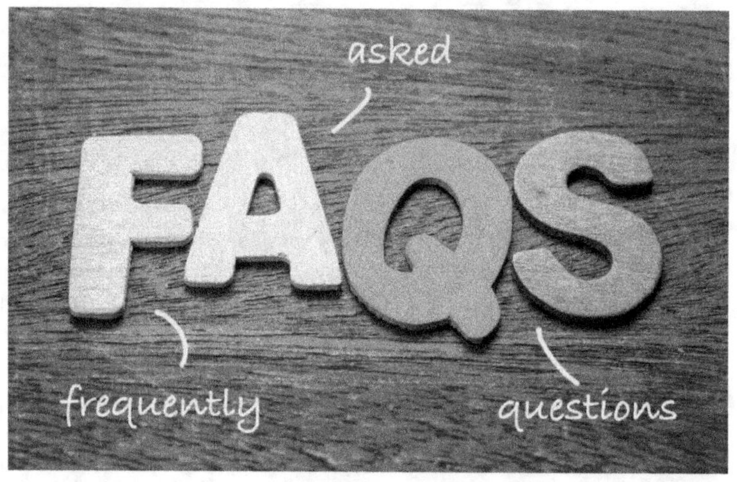

Can I Consume Liquids During the Fasting Period?

Yes. The recommended beverages during your fast are calorie-free drinks, tea, coffee, and water. Do not add sugar to any drink you consume, especially coffee, but scarce amounts of cream or milk may be beneficial. In fact, coffee curbs hunger, which makes it a great idea during fasting periods.

Skipping Breakfast is Unhealthy, Isn't It?

As discussed in chapter two of this section, it is not necessarily unhealthy. When you skip breakfast during intermittent fasting, you will not have to worry too much because you will consume healthy foods throughout the day, anyway. This will balance out your skipped meals because you will have the same amount of calories at differing times of the day.

May I Take Supplements During the Fasting Period?

There is no immediate issue with consuming supplements during your fasting. However, know that most supplements are **fat-soluble**, which means they are more effective when you eat them with a meal.

Is Exercise Recommended During Fasting Periods?

Yes, you can work out during your fasts. It is helpful to take **branched-chain amino acids (BCAAs)** before your workout.

Should My Children Fast?

Doctors do not recommend children perform fasts.

Is Intermittent Fasting Safe for People with Diabetes?

It is safe but will require constant management of your glucose levels, meaning a medical professional will need to supervise you, as you need to ensure that you have the correct medications and insulin levels throughout the process.

If you have type 2 diabetes, you will need to discuss the timing and protocol of your dosages if plan on fasting during the morning hours. Discuss as well about conducting some basal testing so you know how to adjust your personal doses of insulin when required, even if you do not plan on doing extensive fasting. This process is important for overall diabetes management and including if you plan to skip a meal. You will also need to check your blood sugar levels throughout the day to manage it. You will notice a difference in the amount of insulin that you will require within the first few weeks, so checking your blood sugar is important.

Why Should I Fast for 24 Hours?

Fasting for longer hours can help amplify the many health benefits you experience. It allows your body to continue to burn fat cells in your body, and you will see results more quickly.

Am I Going to Gain Back All the Weight I Lost?

This is depends solely on you. If you stop intermittent fasting, you can go back to your old eating habits if you would like. You also have the choice to continue eating healthy meals and exercising regularly. If you want to keep the results of all your hard work, it is likely you will need to choose the latter.

I Like to Exercise. Can I Do This While Fasting?

Yes, but you will not want to do any heavy workouts. If you do, you will wear out your body much faster. The prime time for exercising is right before the fasting period ends. Not only is it a great way to finish your long stretch, but you will also refuel your body healthily to build up your muscles.

Can I Take a Break from Intermittent Fasting?

Yes, it is possible to take a break, and it is the beauty of using intermittent fasting because you can work it around your lifestyle. However, if you plan to go back into intermittent fasting, continue the good eating habits that you were doing before so you do not counteract your hard work up to that point.

Chapter Summary

- Drink water during your fasting period. It serves many functions such as flushing out your system, keeping yourself hydrated, and it will keep you feeling fuller.
- Sometimes you need to take vitamins and supplements to make sure your body is receiving the nourishment that it requires. It is also acceptable to take these supplements during fasting times, but it is better overall to take them with a meal.
- It is okay to take a break from intermittent fasting. Listen to your body to know when the time is right. There are many people who use the intermittent fasting methods often as a maintenance to keep themselves in shape after they have reached their weight loss goals.

In the next chapter, you will read testimonials from other people who have tried the program and about the positive side effects from keeping up with intermittent fasting.

Part Three: Incentives and Risks of Intermittent Fasting

Chapter 1: Intermittent Fasting for Weight Loss and Fighting Diseases

Scientific Studies

There are so many benefits that you can realize when following with intermittent fasting. There are various interesting studies on health conditions, and the most well-known benefit of intermittent fasting is that you can lose weight. People have proven this fact time and time again. A systematic review from forty different studies to show that intermittent fasting reduced participants' body weights[52, 61].

But the benefits do not just stop at losing weight. It causes a ripple effect with other ailments which you can experience within your body on a physical level, also affecting your psyche.

One study conducted by researchers at the University of Alabama used a small test group of obese men who were all diagnosed with prediabetes. Researchers put them onto a **time-restricted feeding regimen**. They split the men into two groups:

> **Group 1:** Eat for eight hours between 7am and 3pm.

> **Group 2:** Eat for twelve hours between 7am and 7pm.

For the first four weeks, there was no loss or gain in weight. However, during the fifth week, Group 1 had lowered their insulin levels a significant amount and dramatically improved their insulin sensitivity. They also saw a significant drop in their blood pressure[59].

A further review into the study of diabetes and the effects of intermittent fasting concluded that fasting can lower insulin levels and blood glucose in people at risk with diabetes. The researchers concluded it resulted from the weight loss which lowered the overall risk for diabetes[1].

You can even improve your triglycerides, cholesterol, heart rate, and blood pressure if you take part in intermittent fasting, according to another study[33].

Some animal studies done on rats have also proven positive for intermittent fasting. For one study, researchers placed a group of mice on an intermittent fasting diet, while researchers allowed the other group full free access to food. The results showed the intermittent fasting mice came out with better memory and learning capabilities than the free access mice[27]. In another study, a suppression in the inflammation within the brain appeared when researchers subjected the animals to an intermittent fasting regimen[62]. This was a significant finding because brain inflammation has links to several neurological conditions.

Further studies using mice also showed a reduced risk of stroke, Parkinson's disease, and Alzheimer's disease. There has even been preliminary findings for the reduction in growth for tumors. They concluded that the reduction in weight was one of the main reasons for this result[33].

One other study focused on the 16:8 Pattern showed a lowered systolic blood pressure in just a few months[9].

As you can see, there is scientific evidence backing up intermittent fasting's ability to not only lower body weight, but also to help the body become a fighting machine against some of the most prevalent diseases in modern society. Hear what some people talk about their experiences and the effects that intermittent fasting has done for them.

Testimonials

"In 7.5 months I've dropped 50 pounds, 10.5% in body fat and 40 inches around my body. These results are entirely as a result of Intermittent Fasting as I was unable to exercise for the first several months due to a fractured foot."[21]

"My weight loss wasn't fast—I was dropping pounds steadily but very slowly. Dealing with this was the hardest part and trying to find the motivation to keep going when my patience was wearing thin was so difficult. But the more I exercised and ate right, the better I felt, and I finally realized that I didn't have to lose five pounds a week to be improving my health (and in fact, it was probably better that I wasn't!). It took me three years, but by 2015, I had lost 90 pounds."[37]

"In two-and-a-half months, I was able to stop all medications and:

- Lowered my HbA1c from 73 mmol/mol to 40 mmol/mol.
- Lowered my weight from 74 kg (163 lbs) to 65 kg (143 lbs) plus added muscle.
- Lowered my waist circumference from 97 cm (38 inches) to 86 cm (34 inches)."[48]

"All of the success stories and research couldn't be wrong about fasting. I eased into 16:8 over a couple of days and by the 10th day on 16:8 I had lost 4 lbs. But more than that, I felt good. More energy, less bloating, and the heart burn I'd started getting most days had gone. Over the following 3 weeks I lost 8 lbs and several inches, and I felt amazing. I increased to 18:6 as wasn't feeling hungry at 16 hrs. It has been 10 months now. I'm down 37 lbs, my blood pressure is back to normal, heartburn gone, resting pulse dropped by 10 points, and I'm in my goal size!"[55]

Chapter Summary

- Several scientific studies on rats and humans show positive results for following the intermittent fasting methods.
- You can see a decrease in blood pressure, cholesterol levels, and insulin levels when using intermittent fasting methods; these benefits are linked to the weight loss that people experience while they are intermittent fasting.
- People have been able to diminish their diabetes medications and see a massive improvement in their health within months; they can lose massive amounts of weight as long as they focus on their aspirations and their personal goals.

In the next chapter, you will learn more about the benefits and risks to intermittent fasting with diabetes, and specific ways that patients can use intermittent fasting to improve their health and reduce the amount of medication they need to live a higher quality of life.

Chapter 2: Intermittent Fasting for Diabetes

During the fasting periods, your body uses the glycogen in the liver as energy. While this process happens, it gives the **pancreas**, the organ that produces insulin, a rest and stops producing new insulin in the body.

According to the American Diabetes Association (ADA), if you have diabetes and is suffering from obesity, you could lower your A1c levels and your risk for heart disease when you lose weight.

The results of one study conducted with mice found that pancreatic fat lowered during intermittent fasting[45]. The study suggests that there is a correlation between a fatty pancreas leading to developing type 2 diabetes. Even if you are at risk of diabetes, implementing intermittent fasting will lower your risk for developing diabetes.

When starting with an intermittent fasting plan, those with type 1 diabetes can lower their insulin dosage. Therefore, if you have type 1 diabetes, it is of utmost importance to be working with your medical professional about going through with intermittent fasting because you will need monitoring and adjustments to your insulin and medications.

There are risks involved when fasting when suffering from diabetes. The biggest danger is you may develop **hypoglycemia**, where blood sugar levels drop to extremely low levels. The symptoms include shakiness throughout the body, passing out, or going into a coma.

Hypoglycemia is most often seen with those taking insulin to control their diabetes because the medications lower insulin levels. During fasting, your body will not be producing insulin, so a medical professional will need to monitor you closely.

There is also a risk when you complete your fasting period to go into hyperglycemia, in which your blood sugar levels would go to the opposite extreme. This condition is a concern if you consume too many carbohydrates, so you would need to avoid them if you have diabetes.

Your doctor will recommend the best course of action for you. If you find that you are having signs of hypoglycemia during your fasting periods, stop the fast and consume a drink containing sugar. When your symptoms subside, eat a small, nutrient-rich meal.

Be sure not to exercise too much during fasting periods. This will cause your blood sugar levels to drop which will put your more at risk for hypoglycemia. Ask for advice from your doctor on which activities are acceptable during your fasting period or refrain from exercise altogether during fasts.

Some studies have researched into how intermittent fasting can help those with both types of diabetes, showing promising results. In one study, researchers investigated three subjects between the ages of ten to 25-years-old who had type 2 diabetes. They fasted for three full days a week for a month. Results showed that all three were able to stop taking insulin, and within a year, were medication-free for their diabetes[8].

Another study done in New Zealand showed that fasting periods increased the risk of hypoglycemia, which was an expected outcome. However, they also saw the subjects had weight loss and a drop in their A1c levels[53].

Here are some suggestions on how to manage your blood sugar levels while you are in your fasting period after you wake up:

If your blood sugar levels are high: Take a reduced correction dose of insulin, given that you know your own correction dose. You will then be able to carry on with the fast. However, by introducing insulin, your body may switch back to burning glucose for fuel.

If you find that this is a regular occurrence, it may have to become part of your normal routine during fasting periods. You must be more gentle with your body during the adjustments and know that they will continue to change throughout the process of intermittent fasting. It is important that you do not create a heightened blood glucose level; you will need to monitor it properly.

If you decide not to take the reduced correction dose of insulin, you will spend the rest of your fasting time with high blood sugar, which is a situation that is not ideal to your overall health. So, keep in mind that your priority will be to ensure your blood sugar levels are within the proper range, even if it switches your body out of fat-burning mode.

If your blood sugar levels are low: You will need to break your fast so you can fuel your metabolism. The fast is not effective in burning fat, so it is best to regulate your blood sugar. Continue with the normal routine for your eating window and do not use the low blood sugar levels as an excuse to overeat. Be sure to eat a sensible meal not loaded with carbohydrates so you do not cause the absolute opposite effect to your blood sugar. Be calm and start again with the process.

Monitor if it becomes a routine to wake up with either too high or too low blood sugar; if you are finding a consistent pattern, you may need to take a hard look at the foods you are consuming before you go on your fast or before you go to sleep in the evening. You will probably need to adjust what you are eating. Do not eat a heavy meal before your eating window finishes. Pay special attention to any carbohydrates you are consuming, as there may be an imbalance between them and the insulin levels. Talk with your doctor about basal testing so you can find a solution to this issue.

Chapter Summary

- With a doctor's supervision, patients can lose weight successfully while reducing their need for medical treatment for diabetes.
- If you find that your blood sugars are too low or high during your fast, take a reduced booster of insulin to regulate your blood sugars. Do not fret if you need to end your fast earlier, as your health is always the most important.
- Use trial-and-error if you are find consistent issues with your glucose levels during fasting periods.

Know that your numbers will fluctuate over time because of the changes in your body.

In the next chapter you will learn about how intermittent fasting can help people with heart conditions.

Chapter 3: Intermittent Fasting for Heart Health

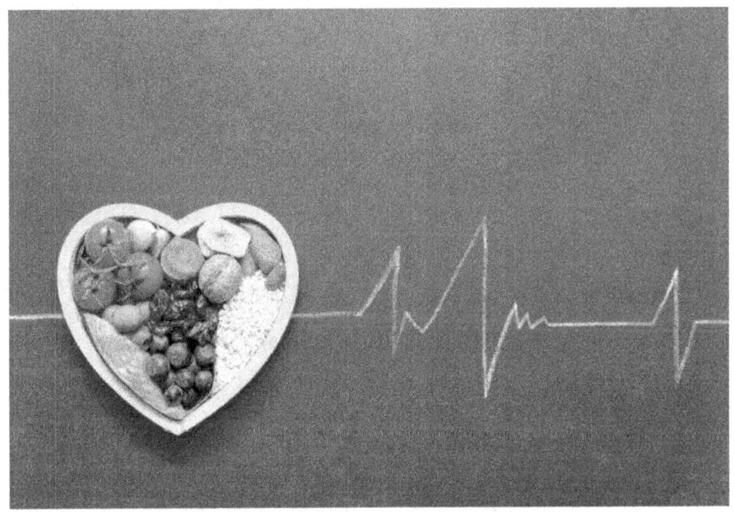

Those suffering from high blood pressure and heart disease can see some benefits to intermittent fasting. The fasting process changes how the body metabolizes sugar and cholesterol, and helps with both issues.

When you fast regularly, you change the way your body uses sugar. You will then lose weight, putting less strain on your heart. Intermittent fasting will also lower your chances for developing diabetes, which is also a risk factor for heart disease.

The same goes for those with heart disease — they will need to consult with their health professional so the latter can properly monitor the individual throughout the process. Because every person's situation is different, you will need to come up with a personal plan for exercise and proper foods to incorporate into your diet while you are in your eating window.

The four heavy hitters for heightening the risk of heart disease are weight issues, diabetes, cholesterol, and high blood pressure. If you can reduce these factors, you will be at a lower risk for heart disease. Luckily, intermittent fasting tackles all these issues, so it can be an excellent option for those battling with heart disease.

There are always risks involved, and it is no different for those with heart-related issues. You should first consult with your physician before starting any change in your lifestyle. Also, during the fasting period, it is possible for an electrolyte imbalance to occur, which can lead to the heart being unstable and causing **arrhythmias.**

To counteract this side effect, you will need to be sure to schedule regular monthly visits to your doctor so they can check your blood pressure levels and prescribe *potassium supplements* to balance out the electrolytes in your system.

Studies on the effects regarding intermittent fasting and heart disease have shown positive results. Various studies concluded that that those who incorporate intermittent fasting in their routine showed to have a much lowered risk at developing heart disease or a stroke[29].

Researchers concluded that the 5:2 diet is the best intermittent fasting method in lowering the amount of fat present in the bloodstream.

During the process, toxins and fat are removed from the bloodstream at a much quicker rate compared to regular eating. Patients also have a much greater reduction in systolic blood pressure when they used this intermittent fasting method.

The actual results were a nine percent reduction in systolic blood pressure for those who followed the 5:2 method compared to a two percent increase for those who did not follow a fasting regimen.

Chapter Summary

- Just like with diabetics, patients with heart conditions will need to have regular screenings with their doctor. Intermittent fasting will help them need less medication or eliminate medications altogether.
- Following intermittent fasting will help those with heart disease, those at risk to lower their blood pressure levels, and those with bad cholesterol levels.
- Fat is flushed out of the bloodstream much more efficiently while on intermittent fasting methods. This process lowers your risk for heart attack and stroke.

In the next chapter, you will learn about how intermittent fasting affects your skin and can help grow back hair.

Chapter 4: Intermittent Fasting for Skin and Hair Care

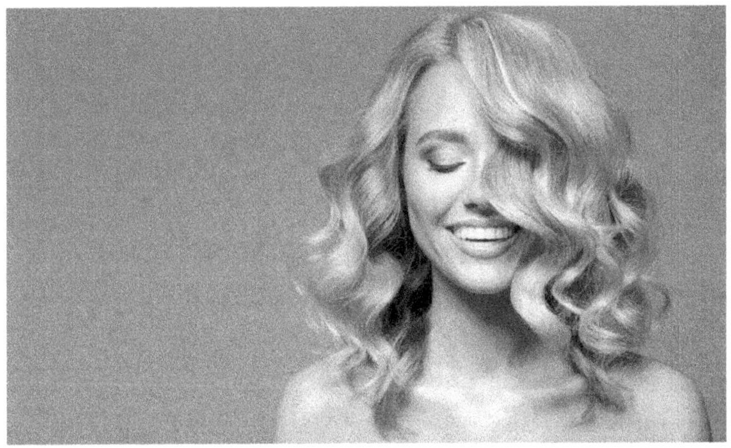

A positive side effect of using intermittent fasting methods is that you will see great improvements in your hair and skin. In fact, one of the current methods to improve hair and skin is through fasting, and you will notice these effects as your skin and hair become more radiant. People usually see these results within weeks of beginning with intermittent fasting methods.

The inside of the body greatly affects the skin, as the skin is the largest organ in the body. Two important components of the skin are proteins known as *collagen* and *elastin*. Protein cells present in the body have a limited lifespan and need to go through a recycling process. During the fasting process, you allow for your body to generate these proteins, which allows your skin to clear up blemishes.

When you want to improve the health of your hair, you will need to use intermittent fasting for a much longer period to see results. In fact, you can even experience temporary hair loss during the process, usually because of the change in hormones, lack of nutrients, calorie deficits, or higher stress levels.

Luckily, these are problems you can tackle for strong hair growth. For stress, pinpoint the source and reduce and eliminate if possible. The rest of the issues focus on having a balanced and nutrient-rich diet and making sure you have the proper amount of calories per day which will aid you in reaching your health goals. In addition, you can incorporate vitamin and mineral supplements as needed.

Chapter Summary

- True beauty comes from within. Once you start the intermittent fasting process, you will clean out the toxins within your body. This cleaning of toxins will cause your skin to glow after a few weeks.
- Even though it is possible to lose hair during intermittent fasting, over time, your hair will grow back thicker than before.
- Hair loss is usually associated with stress and calorie deficits. Ensure that you are consuming enough food during your eating period and that you are keeping your stress levels as low as possible to prevent any calorie deficits.

In the next chapter, you will learn about the specifics of intermittent fasting and women. You will learn more about the best types of intermittent fasting methods for women and also advice for pregnant and breastfeeding mothers.

Chapter 5: Intermittent Fasting for Women

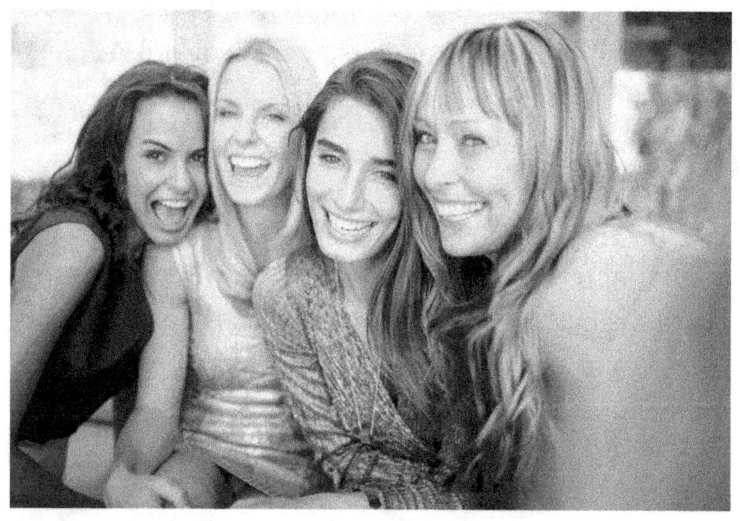

There are differences in how women need to approach intermittent fasting compared to men. As discussed before, there are differing effects that intermittent fasting protocols have on women's bodies, such as blood sugar levels worsening rather than getting better. The good news is that there has been research into this subject, and there are ways to counteract these possibilities.

It is best for women to keep to short timings for fasting, meaning women should begin their intermittent fasting journey by starting with an eight to twelve hour fast. Choose an amount you are comfortable with and then build it by an hour each day. Do not go over 24 hours until you know how the fasts will affect you.

Another concern is the calorie restricted diets. Unfortunately, women's bodies can be to these restrictions, which results in the hypothalamus part of the brain becoming imbalanced. The helper hormone known as **gonadotropin-releasing hormone (GnRH)** is disrupted, which causes a chain reaction. Your body needs the gonadotropin-releasing hormone to secrete two reproductive hormones known as **luteinizing hormone (LH)** and **follicle-stimulating hormone (FSH)**[34, 35].

Because these hormones are not being released, it can cause a pause or a complete stop in a woman's menstrual cycle because the body is not producing estrogen or progesterone to release an egg. This occurrence may not always be the case with all women; However, if you find that you are consistently late or missing periods, you need to consider reviewing your diet and cutting back on your fasting days or periods until your body returns maintenance mode through intermittent fasting[63].

There is scientific evidence to show that short periods of fasting will not affect milk production in breastfeeding mothers; however, you need to be diligent in consuming copious amounts of water. If you become dehydrated, your milk supplies may likely suffer[46].

As for pregnant women, it is better to refrain from intermittent fasting during any part of the pregnancy, including during attempted conception as it will cause harm to the pregnancy during the process. Start the process by eliminating any unhealthy foods and habits out of your life. Once you give birth, you are safe to start the intermittent fasting methods. If you already practiced cutting out unhealthy foods, you will also be more prepared

Teenage girls can benefit from performing intermittent fasting plans. Not only is it easy for a teenager to follow, but there is no reason they should not try fasting for specific amounts at a time. Intermittent fasting can prove helpful for those falling into the overweight bracket, as they will see much worse consequences down that road. If they continue to live their life overweight, they may be prone to major diseases at a younger age. The alternative is for them to start a reduced-calorie diet for a set time.

The catch to this is that they still need to follow a balanced diet which would include whole foods and nutrients. As an example, if there is a deficit in zinc, a child may have stunted growth. If you find the teen may not be receiving the vitamins and minerals they require, you will need to supply them with supplements or add a multivitamin to their diet regimen.

The length of a fast needs to be for about five to six hours; there is no need to go overboard with teenagers. Shifting the first meal of the day until lunchtime, the teenager will see the benefits of being on this altered intermittent fasting method.

Chapter Summary

- Women need to take a much more gentle approach to intermittent fasting because their bodies can have different reactions to restricted diets.
- It is possible for a breastfeeding woman to perform intermittent fasting methods. The key is to consume a large amount of water so you do not reduce your milk production. You should still do this as directed by a medical professional.

- Teenagers can do a modified form of intermittent fasting to help them keep their weight under control and to help them lose weight. Special attention needs to be toward their diet to make sure they are receiving the correct amount of nutrients in their food.

In the next chapter, you will learn about an exercise routine that you can use every day to maximize your results during your intermittent fasting routine.

Chapter 6: Get the Most Out of Intermittent Fasting

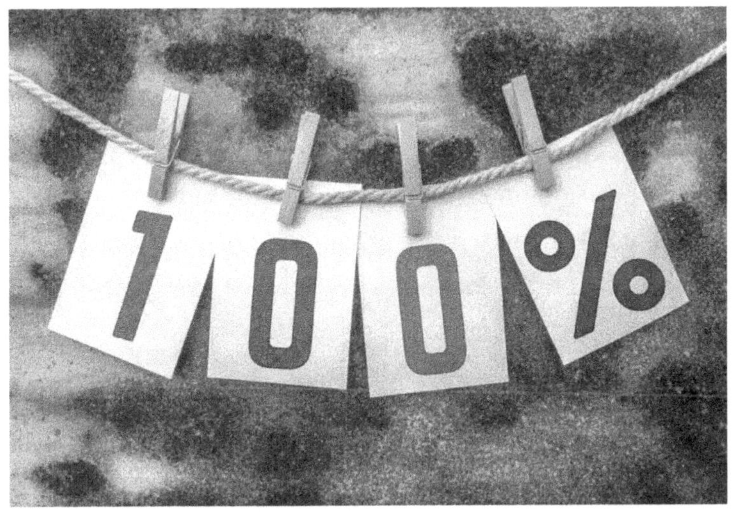

When you want to reach your goals for weight loss, the best way is to set up an exercise routine and couple it with your intermittent fasting method. This can be any non-strenuous activity, as you will need to be gentle to your body while you are in fasting mode. Read some tips before going into the example exercise routine you can incorporate into your day.

Use Your Whole Body

Doing some full-body and balanced exercises aids you to lose more fat, increase your energy levels, and build lean muscle mass. Some exercises that can use both your legs and upper body are **squats** and **lunges**.

Find a Buddy to Exercise With You

When you have another teammate to help motivate you, it will keep you more driven toward your goals. They will also be on the lookout for if you are pushing too hard through your fasting period.

Take a Walk

This suggestion may seem obvious, but people forget how much this simple exercise will benefit your whole body. When you schedule a walk into your daily exercise routine, you increase your focus, improve your recovery time and blood flow, reduce stress, and become leaner.

Why is Warm-Up Important?

It is imperative that you prepare your body for exercise because it will not only minimize the risk of injury, but there is also a purpose for the warm-up exercises.

1. *Increase Your Body Temperature*: By warming up your body, you are widening your range of motion by making your muscles more elastic; this elasticity will help your body perform movements easier and lessen your chances for injury. Performing warm-up exercises will also oxygenate your blood.

2. *Expansion of Blood Vessels*: An expansion in your blood vessels will reduce the risk of high blood pressure during the exercise routine.

3. Your body will produce hormones as your body warms up. These hormones will increase your energy levels during your workout.

Why is it Important to Cool Down After a Workout?

The purpose of the cool-down period is to allow your body to adjust by slowing your heart rate down to the normal rate. The cool-down is an important step in working out because you are more prone to cardiovascular problems just after a workout. You can minimize stiffness and soreness when you perform cool-down exercises, as it helps work out lactic acid that accumulates in your body during exercise. A cool-down session also gives your body a chance to recirculate blood and oxygen.

Warm-Up

To warm your body, you need to use **dynamic stretches** to improve your performance, strength, and power during your exercise routine. These stretches are not isolated where you would stand or sit — these stretches make you move and help better circulate the blood in your bloodstream. There are five stretches that are best to prepare your body for your workout. Be sure to drink plenty of water beforehand so you do not become dehydrated. You should finish *one round* of each exercise before you start any workout:

1. ***Leg Swings***: Hold on to a support such as a bar or a wall and lift one leg out to the side. Then, swoop your leg down across your body to the front of your other leg. Repeat ten times and then switch to the other leg.

2. *Frankenstein Walk*: Tighten and straighten your knees, then walk back and forth while keeping your legs straight, kicking your leg up and reaching for it with your opposite hand with each step. Flex your toes as you walk for fifteen yards.

3. *Walking Lunges*: Step forward with one foot and slowly lower your whole body while dropping your opposite knee toward the ground. Do not let your front knee reach past a 90-degree angle with your front foot. Repeat this step while stepping forward with your other foot for about fifteen yards.

4. *Bent Torso Twists*: Stand with your feet shoulder-width apart and stretch your arms out to the sides. Keep your arms straight out to the sides, then reach down (arms still straight) to touch the opposite foot, other hand reaching toward the sky. While bent down, be sure to keep your back straight with your shoulder blades pushed back. Rotate your core so your other hand touches its opposite foot. Rotate back and forth for twenty repetitions.

5. *Deep Squats*: Stand with your feet shoulder-width apart. Lift your arms in front of your torso; you may either cross your arms, hold them out, or hold them in a "boxing" position. Squat as close as you can to a 90-degree angle while pushing your buttocks out behind you. While in this position, keep your knees behind your toes. Stand back up. Repeat this for ten repetitions.

These exercises should take you anywhere from five to ten minutes to complete. Once you have completed one set of each warm-up exercise, you are ready to move on to your main exercise routine which can include walking, a short jog, roller skating, or another low-cardio workout you enjoy.

Cool-Down Process

Use these exercises to cool your body down after a workout:

1. *Light Jog*: It is always a good idea to try a light five-minute jog after a workout, as it will help flush out lactic acid buildup. Do not run go as hard as you would normally — exaggerate your arm and leg movements and make them move, but go slow.

2. *Lunging Hip Flexor Stretch*: Set your feet slightly less than shoulder-width apart. Step forward with one foot so it is flat on the floor,

then extend your arms upward; your other food should be bent. Keep your torso and hips straight and squat down, pressing your hips down and forward. Hold the position for five seconds, then stand up straight while lowering your arms. Repeat a few times with on both sides.

3. *Seated Hamstring Stretch*: Sit on the floor with your knees straight and your legs apart at a 45-degree angle in front of you. Reach with both hands toward one foot while keeping your back straight. Hold for 20 seconds and repeat with the other leg.

4. *Shoulder Stretch*: Lift one arm over your head and bend it at the elbow. Press your bent arm toward the center of your back and press on it gently with the other hand. Move the same arm across your torso so it extends across your chest and press the elbow joint gently with the other hand. Hold for 20 seconds, then repeat this stretch with the other arm.

At the end of your workout routine, go home, take a shower, and give yourself a good night's sleep. If you are doing your routine right before the end of your fasting period, have a sensible snack and then have a good meal one or two hours after the workout. Remember to drink plenty of water to keep hydrated!

Chapter Summary

- It is important to set up an exercise routine that is not too strenuous so you can maximize your results in intermittent fasting.
- You need to make sure you stretch out your muscles ahead of your workout because your muscles will be more elastic to lessen your chances of injury.
- Be sure to stay hydrated throughout your workout. Because you are also fasting, you will need to drink more water than you think you may need.

In the next chapter, you will learn how to follow intermittent fasting methods safely. These tips will help you in the long run and aid in case you find yourself in a difficult situation.

Chapter 7: Precautions during Intermittent Fasting

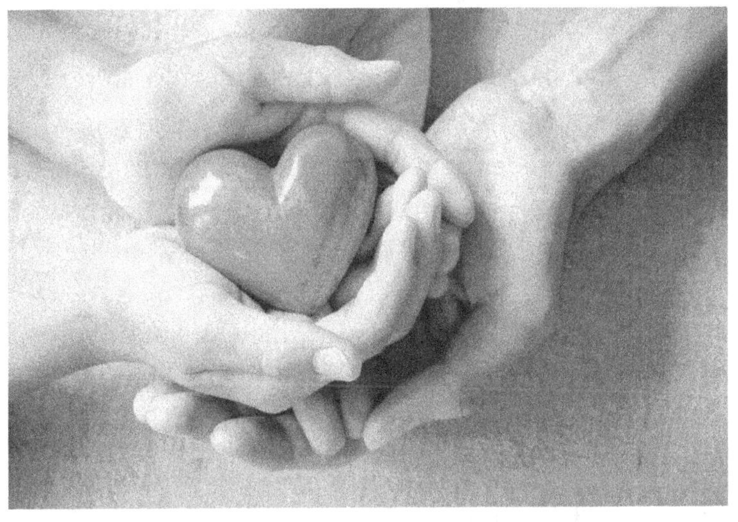

While implementing intermittent fasting into your life, it is important to take precautions so you can stay safe during the process. You need to respect your body and what it tries to tell you at all times. For example, if you feel ill, dizzy, lightheaded, or something does not seem right, it may be best to break your fast early. Your health is the number one priority here, and there is nothing wrong with breaking a fast if it is in the best interest of your health. Do not let pride get in the way. Hunger pains, however, are not a good enough reason to stop the fasting process.

At first, you will want to keep your fasting periods short, especially if you have never done a fast before. This will help you notice how your body reacts to the fasting process, and you can build your perseverance in baby steps. Even if you need to fast for eight hours, you need to do what you know you can to accomplish your goal. Once you achieve these small baby steps, you will have more confidence in yourself and your body to make it through another hour or two the next day. Always push yourself, but not too far as to risk your health.

The longer the fasting period, the more attention you will need to put toward drinking plenty of water. This will help the process move much smoother for you. You can drink sparkling water, tea, and coffee during your fast; however, you will want to limit your caffeinated drinks to three during your fasting period. Otherwise, the caffeine may have a negative effect on your body.

Other issues which can arise the longer you perform the fast are an inability to focus, lack of energy, hunger pains, fainting, mood swings, and irritability[7, 11, 50]. If you find that you have these issues often during your fasting period, you need to observe what you are eating before you enter a fast, or try to shorten your fasting periods until your body adjusts to the changes. Remember that the fasting process needs to be gradual.

You can also eat a restricted diet on your fasting days while you work toward longer periods. This strategy will assist your body in the transition and build you up to the partial fast while also drinking water. You should eat small snacks equating to 500 calories for women and 600 calories for men. Once you have introduced the restricted diet on fasting days for about a week, cut back to the partial fast for optimal benefits.

Water is of utmost importance. If you are not drinking enough water when you are fasting, you will go through symptoms of dehydration, which include headaches, thirst, dry mouth, and fatigue. Dehydration can occur much quicker than usual during the fasting process, so it is best to continue as much as you can during the fasting period[44]. Health professionals recommend that people drink roughly eight glasses of eight ounces of water each day. You may find that you need more, and that is fine; the bottom line is that you listen to your body[36].

You also need to watch your mental health during a fast. When you are not used to fasting, it can seem like it is dragging on forever, which is the case when you mind is constantly thinking about food and when you can eat again. Try to keep your mind on more important things. When you keep your thoughts in check, the fasting experience can be a time that you would use to become more in touch with your inner self. Take the time to meditate to clear your mind of these thoughts; the time will pass quicker when you are in a positive state of mind.

You do not have to meditate if you do not want to — you can engage in any activity that is not too strenuous to keep your mind occupied. As long as it is something you enjoy, the time will fly by. Think about catching up on that book you have been meaning to read or take some me time by taking a long and relaxing bath.

One dangerous pitfall is that it is tempting to gorge yourself once you come off of your fast. You will want to congratulate yourself for making it through your fast, but try to avoid celebrating with food, as you will only complicate matters if you eat a large meal after completing your fast. Lots of food at once will make you feel tired and bloated, and it will be harder to do your next fast. From a caloric standpoint, you set yourself up to consume excessive calories because you will want to eat further along in your eating window. The best solution is to start off with a small snack or sensible meal when you enter back into your eating window. This approach will eliminate the feelings of hunger, and you will not have to suffer through an upset stomach.

If you eat enough protein during your eating windows, you will not only gain the energy you need to get through the day, but it will help you also build muscle mass. Because you work on an overall calorie deficit, you could also lose some muscle mass. When you counterbalance this deficit with a sufficient amount of proteins, you will see your muscles grow[5, 7].

If you do a restricted diet on your fasting days, you will feel less hungry when consuming proteins as part of your diet. A study concluded that approximately 30% of your calories come from proteins, meaning that a restricted diet will help you reduce your hunger cravings[26].

When you want to be safe while supplying your body with the nutrients it needs, supplements will be something to consider. Because you are restricting your caloric intake, you may not consume all the vitamins and minerals that your body needs. The nutrients that hit the heaviest during intermittent fasting are vitamin B12, calcium, and iron[4]. If you are worried that there may be other nutrients that you are not receiving, a multivitamin can cover it. However, even though it may be easy to take a supplement or multivitamin, it is best for your body to consume the nutrients you require through whole foods. So, do not fall into the trap of taking a multivitamin and only focusing on a few food groups[18].

Chapter Summary

- Water is the most important aspect during your fasting period. The second most important are your thought processes. You will want to keep a positive frame of mind throughout the fasting process.
- If feel ill or faint during the fasting period, break the fast with a small snack. This should help you feel better. You can try again the next day.
- Some people will find they cannot receive all of their nutrients from the foods they eat. One way to solve this is to take supplements or a multivitamin to bridge the gap, but do not take these as a complete alternative.

In the next chapter, you will learn about the downsides to intermittent fasting, and what you can do to counteract them.

Chapter 8: The Downside of Intermittent Fasting

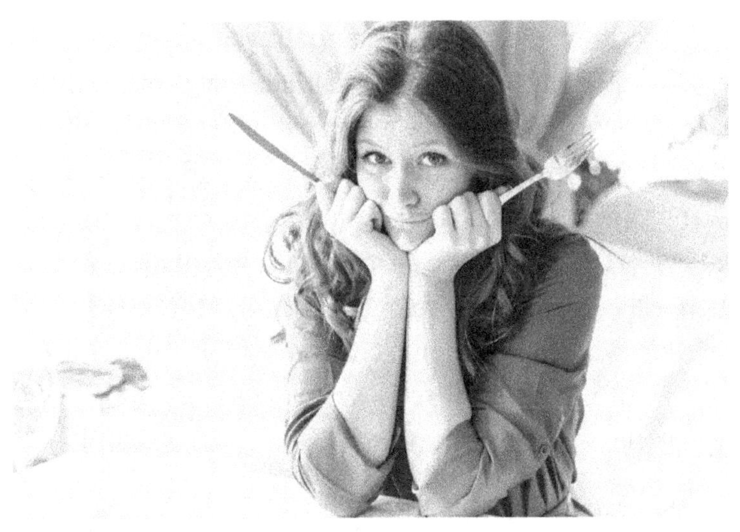

You are likely to feel hungry during your fasting period. However, there are several ways you can counteract this feeling. If you follow just a few steps, then you will know how to move through your fasting period easier without enduring constant hunger pains the whole time.

First, look at whether you have chosen the correct intermittent fasting method for you, or if you maybe one that's a little too much for you to handle. You may have been confident in starting with the full blown 16 hours or more for your first time; however, starting at 12 hours and building up to more hours of fasting is more efficient, and you will feel less hungry during the process.

It is also helpful to eat the foods you enjoy at first and then slowly incorporate healthier foods into your diet. It is more helpful if you can cut out the sugar and high carbohydrates from the beginning, but you do not want to shock your system by making too many changes at first. You will find the process much more difficult, and you will be more likely to quit intermittent fasting because you will not think it is working for you. Be sure to look at portion control as well so you can see the weight loss benefits faster.

You should drink a full glass of water to help curve your hunger pains. This is because your body becomes dehydrated while you sleep, and coupled with the fasting periods, your body will crave water. It also revs up the organs in your body so they can work through the day. Aim for drinking 16 ounces of water first thing after you wake up, and you will notice the hunger cravings subsiding.

With fasting, willpower is the key. You will need to push through some tough times, and you will need the motivation to succeed. Have a pep talk with yourself when you are feeling low. You need to remind yourself why you are fasting in the first place and rise above the problems. When you can switch your thinking and empower yourself to push through, you are halfway through the battle.

If you keep yourself busy doing other things, you are likely not to notice that you have not eaten for so long. Keeping your mind on tasks will be a healthy distraction. You will see that you won't be looking at your app every five minutes to see how long you have left in the fasting period as often, and it will help you be more productive when you can shift your focus to something else.

If you still feel hungry, make yourself a cup of flavored tea. The flavoring of your fruit or herbal tea will trick your mind into thinking you are giving it something to satisfy your hunger. It will also add some variety from drinking plain water during your fast. It is also wise to find a sugarless gum that you enjoy when you are feeling hunger pains. The motion of your mouth chewing triggers a psychological response to your hunger. Be sure you do not consume any other sweets such as candies, cough drops, or mints, as they are counterproductive to your body's ability to stay in ketones.

Sometimes the reason you feel excessively hungry is that you may not be consuming the right foods during your eating window, or you are not eating enough to nourish your body. Although many people say you can eat whatever you wish during your eating periods, it is counterproductive for you to do so during your fasting period. If you eat junk food and candy instead of whole-food meals with a balance of complex carbohydrates, healthy fats, and protein, you will be sluggish and as a result, the fasting experience will be more difficult.

Be sure you are resting your body each night by getting a good night's sleep. Sleep will help you rejuvenate your body while it is goes through the changes that come with fasting, and it will help you become more aware and energized during the day. If you do not get enough sleep, there will be an overload of the hormone **ghrelin**, which signals to your body that you are hungry.

If you find you are exhausted often, you may be overdoing the intermittent fasting process and your body is playing catch up. This is when you need to know your limits; it is healthy to push the envelope of your boundaries, but it is best to let your body work in the changes before doing so.

Sometimes, the intermittent fasting lifestyle is too much, and in these situations, it is alright to take a small break. This way, you will have time to evaluate what worked and what did not work so you can tackle intermittent fasting from a different angle and with a different attitude. If you struggle with your relationship with food, you may find this to be the case. You need to look at where you are and where you want to go in terms of your goals. Once you have a better idea of your goals and how to get there, then you can use intermittent fasting to help you get there.

Many people go through mood swings while they are in intermittent fasting. When blood sugar levels drop, brain function also falls along with it, which is likely the source for these mood swings. This can lead to an emotional response of being crabby when in fact is it just a reaction to the physical response of fasting.

You will find yourself on an emotional rollercoaster when you have a negative or dependent relationship with food. If your day centered around food before, you may feel anxious when you can no longer eat when you would like. You may feel out of control; however, you can always control how you react and respond to stimuli.

Other people may not realize the actual effects that intermittent fasting will have on them. They may have had a fantasized view of it being easy and found out the hard way that such is not always the case. Remember your personal goals and know that they will require a significant amount of hard effort, but despite whatever it takes, you will reach them. With this mindset, nothing will get in your way.

As your body shifts with intermittent fasting, you may experience headaches more frequently. It is a common occurrence and should not alarm you, as it is how your body initially reacts to the change in your eating schedule. Dehydration could also be a factor, so whenever your head hurts, drink a glass of water to see if it subsides. It also can be because of stress — are you worrying too much about intermittent fasting or are there other things in your life contributing to your headache? If the latter is the case, take a few deep breaths and return your focus to the task at hand. Stress is not an added component that will help you with intermittent fasting, so it is best to keep it at a minimum if possible.

During the first few weeks of intermittent fasting, you will probably be low in energy. This is a sign from your body that you may be exerting too much energy on activities. Be sure to listen to your body during this period of transition. Not only will you make it easier for yourself, but it is healthy for you to take a break for your own wellbeing. If you work out too hard, maybe switch to doing yoga stretches or going on a walk. These exercises will put less strain on your body while intermittent fasting.

If you can follow these simple tricks, you will have an easier time going through your fasting periods. There will be difficulties, but now you know how to tackle those issues like a pro.

Chapter Summary

- There will be some side effects as your body goes through the shifts of intermittent fasting. This is normal, and there is no reason to drop the program, as there are ways to prevent and push through them.
- Make sure you are getting enough rest at night — your body is like a construction project and it needs to have time to rejuvenate so you can have enough energy for the next day.
- The physical effects you experience have the possible added side effect of making you irritated. During these times, embrace it as part of the process and breathe through it. It will not last forever.

In the next chapter, you will learn how to continue to push yourself to live a better life.

Chapter 9: Better Habits for a Better Life

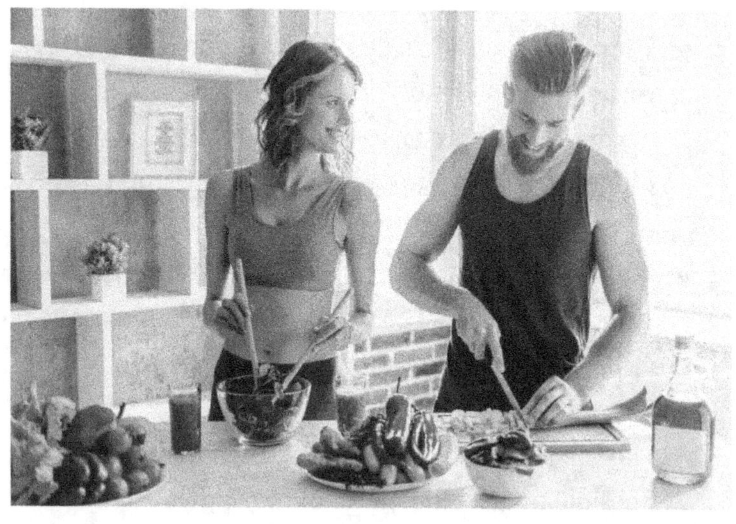

There are always ways in which you can improve your life. You must know the faults you may have and own up to them. In that process, come up with a plan to challenge this part of yourself so you can improve. You need to take charge and make choices every day that will help you improve your life.

It is important to the intermittent fasting process to respect your body. You need to regard your body as a holy place, and something that needs to be revered and worshipped. The better care you take of your body, the longer it will carry you on in life. When this happens, you will have more time to enjoy all the things this world has to offer. So what else can you do today to make yourself or the world around you a better place?

Perhaps you have picked up the habit of smoking. You know that this is bad for your health and you may be addicted. However, even if you strive to smoke a little less each day, you will break that cycle of addiction. It will take some willpower and perseverance, but you can do it. Thousands of people quit every day.

Or maybe you can think about helping your community. You can make small changes that will make a huge impact. One way to impact your community would be to take your own bags to the grocery store. Not only are you recycling, but you are also helping the environment from pollution, and Mother Nature will thank you.

Maybe you need to think about where you spend your money. Instead of going grocery shopping at the big box supermarket, look for deals with your local mom and pop stores and farmers markets. They are your neighbors, and they work very hard. Help to build your community by keeping your hard earned money within the community.

There are other personal ways that you can improve yourself too. You can let go of any hurt or pain that you are holding on from your past, as these are heavy burdens that you can free yourself from. When you can forgive yourself for things you have done and can say sorry, you will notice the weight of it fall off you. You can heal yourself and others in ways that you could not imagine if you put in the effort.

Find appreciation in the people and things that you have in life and then be thankful in things you do not have. When you can see things in this world with this perspective, you will see everything, inside and out, and transform it in beautiful ways. You will sense the possibility in every situation you put yourself into and see the positive side of life. When you view the world as your friend rather than something to fear, you will find that your quality of life will skyrocket.

Keep your heart and mind in the *here* and *now*. It is good to dream about the future, but you must also think of the steps you must take to get to that point. If you do not involve yourself in your life and relationships you have now, you will miss out on some beautiful experiences. Treasure the friends and family that you have in your life and let them know how much you love and appreciate them. Anything can change in an instant, and you do not want to carry any regrets or worries if they know how you perceive them. You will brighten up their day when you do, and you will feel good about it too.

Keep yourself open for any opportunities you may come across, as they are sometimes subtle. When you push yourself out of your comfort zone, much like you are during the intermittent fasting program, you can grow and learn more about yourself. Then you can help others learn the knowledge you have gained through life. You will become a better brother, sister, mother, father, and friend to all of those around you. Always strive to be your best, and wonderful opportunities will come your way.

No matter what point in life you are at, there is always a way that you can improve yourself. You could learn a new language and make new friends around the world; you could volunteer at the local homeless shelter; or you could visit your elderly grandmother and have lunch with her once a week. There are thousands of ways you can touch other people in ways that they will always remember.

Whatever and however you plan to enrich your life, you are always in control of the choices you make. Be sure to make the best choices for yourself and those around you. Change is the nature of the world and is something that we all need to embrace. When we shy away from changes, we miss out on opportunities to grow as a person mentally, physically, and spiritually. However, when we embrace these changes along with all the trials that they may put us through, we can learn so much about ourselves.

When things seem to be at their worst, this is when we can rise above, become stronger, and perhaps learn the lessons we were meant to in this life. The best way to live life is to overcome the obstacles and challenges that life puts in our way. So, now that you are taking on this challenge of intermittent fasting, perceive all the changes in a positive light, and keep your eye on the prize.

Once you realize that you only have one body to get you through life, you will learn to love and respect your body much more. Your body is a temple and you need to treat and maintain it like you would any house of worship — with reverence. To do this, you will need to improve your thinking and your physical health so you can be the absolute best you can be.

If there are any bad habits entangled in you that are keeping you from rising higher, work to make small changes towards fixing the larger issues. The longer a habit has been in place, the harder and longer it will take to break it. The bottom line is that it is possible, and it is up to your attitude and motivation whether or not you complete your goals. You are the only one standing in the way of changing your life. Blaming anyone else for standing in your way is just an excuse.

Take pride in being your individual self and strive to push yourself to new heights. There is always room for improvement within yourself. By reading this book, you are already on a positive track to changing your health. Continue on this path by working at improving yourself a little each day. This change can be something physical, psychological, spiritual, or even learning new things.

Once you take ownership of your life and where you are going, so many opportunities open up for you. When you are more conscious of yourself and your surroundings, you will see everything in a brand new perspective.

Even with our relationships with other people, we can all work to being more empathetic, caring, thoughtful, and supportive. We can rid ourselves of things that will not help us be better people.

We can also think more about our environment around us. When you go shopping, be more conscious about your impact on the world. Bring your own bags to the grocery store and take the time to exercise by riding your bike. You will not only be helping yourself but also the environment.

You should also know where your food comes from. As it was explained before, you can help your community by buying local and supporting mom and pop shops with your money. When you spend your money at big box stores, that money typically goes elsewhere which hurts the people you come in contact with each day.

These little changes you can make in your life will not only help you feel better, but they will also help make great impacts on the world around you. When you can appreciate your environment, you are more willing to continue the cycle doing even more. The longer you keep up with the small changes, the more they become habits, and then they will become who you are at the core and what you base your life on. Always strive to be the best "you" that you can be.

You are the writer of your own destiny. There is no one else who can live your life for you. Embrace the person you are and always work towards improvement, even in small ways. You will realize over time that they build up to magnificent changes. And above all, always celebrate who you are as an individual because you make this world unique.

Final Words

When you incorporate intermittent fasting into your life, you bring opportunities of good health and wellness to your life. It will not happen overnight, and it could take longer than most other people — but it is a journey that you can enjoy as you deepen your relationship with food and yourself.

You have seen first hand the scientific evidence that backs up the claims of millions of people who have gone through intermittent fasting. It is exciting to share all of this new information with you, and they are always uncovering more. When all seems hopeless because you are suffering from overweight problems or other major medical issues, it is easy to feel down. However, there is hope when you use intermittent fasting to change your life.

You now know that it is possible to live your life free of these medical burdens. All it takes is the determination to make your life of higher quality and something you can enjoy. If it helps you, find a role model who has done the same so you can use them as an example for yourself. It is an empowering feeling when you can stop taking a medication that you used to need to live through your day. When you show that you can beat any challenge set forth in front of you, the strength you will gain will carry you through the toughest times in life.

There is no excuse now not to be enthusiastic about this path in your life. There is a real possibility, and it is all in your hands; all you have to do is jump in and trust yourself. Remember that promise in the introduction? You should realize by now the major changes that can occur in your life after you work with the intermittent fasting plan.

Not only are you going to be more energetic, more clear-headed, and maybe even notice you can fight all the diseases in the world, but you will be living a life in a much healthier fashion. You will feel better about yourself for making these lifestyle changes, and then this effect will ripple to the other people you may live with. It will reach out to the people you see in your community and the other people you come in contact with every day.

The possibilities are endless when you can reach your personal goals. If there is nothing else that you get from reading this book, I want you to know that you are capable of living the life that you want and achieving any goals you set out for yourself with intermittent fasting. Only you hold the key to your own happiness, so run after it. You are worth it.

You are in the company of millions of people in the world, including celebrities and movie stars. Most of them have followed the 16:8 pattern, and you can follow in their footsteps. Lance Bass, the famous singer from The Backstreet Boys, swears by the intermittent fasting methods. He said that it seems natural to him now to go on a fast for 12 hours, as it makes him feel healthier and slimmer.

Chris Pratt, the *Jurassic Park* movie star is also giving intermittent fasting a go. He said that he feels great after he starting and also saw some pounds shed. Kate Walsh from *Private Practice* is a well-known face on television. She noticed that people lose water weight before they lose fat, although this is part of the process. She also claimed that it gives her a lot of clarity and energy. Halle Berry, another well-known movie star, looks as if she is going back in time — she attributes her ageless beauty to following the Keto diet and intermittent fasting. She also said that it is good for her mind and body alike.

Even the famed Kourtney Kardashian has gotten into practicing intermittent fasting. She also coupled up intermittent fasting with the Keto diet, and she said that she saw benefits all around with how she felt inside and out. Jimmy Kimmel, who has a late night talk show, claimed that he lost 25 pounds while using intermittent fasting, and has managed to keep the weight off. Hats off to everyone, including yourself, for taking this brave step to changing your life!

References

1. Barnosky, Adrienne R., et al."Intermittent Fasting vs
    Daily Calorie Restriction for Type 2 Diabetes
    Prevention: a Review of Human Findings."
    Translational Research, vol. 164, no. 4, 2014, pp.
    302–311., doi:10.1016/j.trsl.2014.05.013.
2. Burke, Lora E., et al. "Self-Monitoring in Weight
    Loss: A Systematic Review of the Literature."
    Journal of the Academic of Nutrition and Dietetics,
    vol. 111, no. 1, Jan. 30 2012.
    doi:10.1016/j.jada.2010.10.008.
3. Cameron, Jameason D. et al. "Increased Meal
    Frequency Does Not Promote Greater Weight Loss in
    Subjects Who Were Prescribed an 8-week Equi-
    Energetic Energy-Restricted Diet." *British Journal of
    Nutrition*, vol. 103, no. 8, 2009, pp. 1098–1101.,
    doi:10.1017/s0007114509992984.
4. Calton, Jayson B. "Prevalence of Micronutrient
    Deficiency in Popular Diet Plans." *Journal of the
    International Society of Sports Nutrition*, vol. 7, no.
    24, 10 June 2010. doi:10.1186/1550-2783-7-24.

5. Cava, Edda, N. C. Yeat, and B. Mittendorfer. "Preserving Healthy Muscle During Weight Loss." *Advances in Nutrition*, vol. 8, no. 3, 15 May 2017, pp. 511-519. doi:10.3945/an.116.014506.

6. Dhurandhar, Emily J., et al. "The Effectiveness of Breakfast Recommendations on Weight Loss: a Randomized Controlled Trial." *The American Journal of Clinical Nutrition,* vol. 100, no. 2, Apr. 2014, pp. 507–513. doi:10.3945/ajcn.114.089573.

7. Finnell, John S., et al. "Is Fasting Safe? A Chart Review of Adverse Events During Medically Supervised, Water-only Fasting." *BMC Complementary and Alternative Medicine*, vol. 18, no. 67, 20 Feb. 2018. doi:10.1186/s12906-018-2136-6.

8. Furmli, Suleiman, et al. "Therapeutic Use of Intermittent Fasting for People with Type 2 diabetes as an Alternative to Insulin." *British Medical Journal: Case Reports*, Sept. 2018, doi:10.1136/bcr-2017-221854.

9. Gabel, Kelsey, et al. "Effects of 8-Hour Time Restricted Feeding on Body Weight and Metabolic Disease Risk Factors in Obese Adults: A Pilot Study." *Nutrition and Healthy Aging*, vol. 4, no. 4, 2018, pp. 345–353. doi:10.3233/nha-170036.

10. Hartman, M. L., et al. "Augmented Growth Hormone (GH) Secretory Burst Frequency and Amplitude Mediate Enhanced GH Secretion during a Two-Day Fast in Normal Men." *The Journal of Clinical*

Endocrinology & Metabolism, vol. 74, no. 4, Jan. 1992, pp. 757-765. doi:10.1210/jcem.74.4.1548337.

11. Harvie, Michelle, and Anthony Howell. "Potential Benefits and Harms of Intermittent Energy Restriction and Intermittent Fasting Amongst Obese, Overweight and Normal Weight Subjects-A Narrative Review of Human and Animal Evidence." *Behavioral Science*, vol 7, no. 1, 19 Jan. 2017, pp. 4. doi:10.3390/bs7010004.

12. Heilbronn, Leonie K., et al. "Alternate-day Fasting in Nonobese Subjects: Effects on Body Weight, Body Composition, and Energy Metabolism." *The American Journal of Clinical Nutrition*, vol. 81, no. 1, Jan. 2005, pp. 69–73. doi:10.1093/ajcn/81.1.69.

13. Heilbronn, Leonie K., et al. "Glucose Tolerance and Skeletal Muscle Gene Expression in Response to Alternate Day Fasting." *Obesity Research*, vol. 13, no. 3, 2005, pp. 574–581., doi:10.1038/oby.2005.61.

14. Hentry, Tanya A. "Adult obesity rates rise in 6 states, exceed 35% in 7."*American Medical Association,* https://www.ama-assn.org/delivering-care/public-health/adult-obesity-rates-rise-6-states-exceed-35-7.

15. Ho, K. Y., et al. "Fasting Enhances Growth Hormone Secretion and Amplifies the Complex Rhythms of Growth Hormone Secretion in Man." *Journal of Clinical Investigation*, vol. 81, no. 4, Jan. 1988, pp. 968–975., doi:10.1172/jci113450.

16. Hutchison, Amy T., and Leonie K. Heilbronn. "Metabolic Impacts of Altering Meal Frequency and Timing – Does When We Eat Matter?" *Biochimie,*

vol. 124, 2016, pp. 187–197.,
doi:10.1016/j.biochi.2015.07.025.

17. "Diabetes Facts & Figures." *International Diabetes Federation*, https://www.idf.org/aboutdiabetes/what-is-diabetes/facts-figures.html.

18. Jacobs, David R., et al. "Food Synergy: an Operational Concept for Understanding Nutrition." *The American Journal of Clinical Nutrition*, vol. 89, no. 5, 11 Mar. 2009, pp. 1543S-1548S. doi:10.3945/ajcn.2009.26736B.

19. Johnstone, A. M. "Fasting? The Ultimate Diet?" *Obesity Reviews*, vol. 8, no. 3, 2007, pp. 211–222., doi:10.1111/j.1467-789x.2006.00266.x.

20. Johnstone, A. M., et al. "Effect of an Acute Fast on Energy Compensation and Feeding Behaviour in Lean Men and Women." *International Journal of Obesity*, vol. 26, no. 12, 2002, pp. 1623–1628., doi:10.1038/sj.ijo.0802151.

21. Kazi, Sumaya. "My Intermittent Fasting Lifestyle: How I Dropped 50 Pounds." *Medium*, Personal Growth, 23 Aug. 2019, https://medium.com/personal-growth/myifguide-38037b3b1ec4.

22. Kong, Angela, et al. "Self-Monitoring and Eating-Related Behaviors Are Associated with 12-Month Weight Loss in Postmenopausal Overweight-to-Obese Women." *Journal of the Academy of Nutrition and Dietetics*, vol. 112, no. 9, Sept. 2012, pp. 1428-1435. doi:10.1016/j.jand.2012.05.014.

23. Larsson, Susanna C., et al. "Nut Consumption and Incidence of Seven Cardiovascular Diseases." *British*

Medical Journal: Heart, vol. 104, no. 19, 2018, pp. 1615–1620. doi:10.1136/heartjnl-2017-312819.

24. Lee, Kayoung. "Long-Term Weight Loss Maintenance." *The Korean Journal of Obesity*, vol. 24, no. 4, Dec. 2015, pp. 179–183.. doi:10.7570/kjo.2015.24.4.179.

25. Leidy, Heather J., et al. "Effects of Acute and Chronic Protein Intake on Metabolism, Appetite, and Ghrelin During Weight Loss." *Obesity*, vol. 15, no. 5, 6 Sept. 2012. doi:10.1038/oby.2007.143

26. Leidy, Heather J., et al. "The Influence of Higher Protein Intake and Greater Eating Frequency on Appetite Control in Overweight and Obese Men." *Obesity*, vol. 18, no. 9, 2010, pp. 1725–1732. doi:10.1038/oby.2010.45.

27. Li, Liaoliao, et al. "Chronic Intermittent Fasting Improves Cognitive Functions and Brain Structures in Mice." *PLoS ONE*, vol. 8, no. 6, Mar. 2013. doi:10.1371/journal.pone.0066069.

28. Longo, Valter. "Faculty of 1000 Evaluation for Dietary Restriction in Rats and Mice: a Meta-Analysis and Review of the Evidence for Genotype-Dependent Effects on Lifespan." *Biomedical Literature*, 2016. doi:10.3410/f.726086377.793513624.

29. Malinowski, Bartosz, et al. "Intermittent Fasting in Cardiovascular Disorders—An Overview." *Nutrients*, vol. 11, no. 3, 2019, pp. 673. doi:10.3390/nu11030673.

30. Mansell, P. I., et al. "Enhanced Thermogenic
    Response to Epinephrine after 48-h Starvation in
    Humans." *American Journal of Physiology*, vol. 258,
    no. 1, 1 Jan. 1990.
    doi:10.1152/ajpregu.1990.258.1.r87.

31. Martin, Bronwen, et al. "Sex-Dependent Metabolic,
    Neuroendocrine, and Cognitive Responses to Dietary
    Energy Restriction and Excess." *Endocrinology*, vol.
    148, no. 9, 2007, pp. 4318–4333.
    doi:10.1210/en.2007-0161.

32. Martin, Bronwen, et al. "Gonadal Transcriptome
    Alterations in Response to Dietary Energy Intake:
    Sensing the Reproductive Environment." *PLoS ONE*,
    vol. 4, no. 1, July 2009.
    doi:10.1371/journal.pone.0004146.

33. Mattson, Mark P., et al. "Impact of Intermittent
    Fasting on Health and Disease Processes." *Ageing
    Research Reviews*, vol. 39, 2017, pp. 46–58.,
    doi:10.1016/j.arr.2016.10.005.

34. Meczekalski, Blazej, et al. "Functional Hypothalamic
    Amenorrhea and Its Influence on Women's Health."
    Journal of Endocrinological Investigation, vol. 37,
    no. 11, Nov. 2014, pp. 1049-1056.
    doi:10.1007/s40618-014-0169-3.

35. Meczekalski, Blazej, et al. "Functional Hypothalamic
    Amenorrhea: Current View on Neuroendocrine
    Aberrations. *Gynecological Endocrinology*, vol. 1,
    no. 1, 24 Jan. 2008, pp. 4-11,
    doi:10.1080/09513590701807381.

36. Millard-Stafford, Mindy L., et al. "Thirst and Hydration Status in Everyday Life." *Nutrition Reviews*, vol. 70, no. s2, Nov. 2012, pp. S147-S151. doi:10.1111/J.1753-4887.2012.00527.X.

37. Montgomery, Courtney and Charlotte Hilton Anderson. "'Intermittent Fasting Helped Me Lose 90 Pounds.'" Women's Health, Women's Health, 30 Nov. 2018, https://www.womenshealthmag.com/weight-loss/a24268738/courtney-montgomery-intermittent-fasting-weight-loss-success/.

38. Mumme, Karen, and Welma Stonehouse. "Effects of Medium-Chain Triglycerides on Weight Loss and Body Composition: A Meta-Analysis of Randomized Controlled Trials." *Journal of the Academy of Nutrition and Dietetics*, vol. 115, no. 2, 2015, pp. 249–263. doi:10.1016/j.jand.2014.10.022.

39. Munsters, Marjet J. M., and Wim H. M. Saris. "Effects of Meal Frequency on Metabolic Profiles and Substrate Partitioning in Lean Healthy Males." *PLoS ONE*, vol. 7, no. 6, 2012. doi:10.1371/journal.pone.0038632.

40. Nair, K. S., et al. "Leucine, Glucose, and Energy Metabolism after 3 Days of Fasting in Healthy Human Subjects." *The American Journal of Clinical Nutrition*, vol. 46, no. 4, Jan. 1987, pp. 557–562. doi:10.1093/ajcn/46.4.557.

41. Novotny, Janet A., et al. "Discrepancy between the Atwater Factor Predicted and Empirically Measured Energy Values of Almonds in Human Diets." *The

American Journal of Clinical Nutrition, vol. 96, no. 2, Mar. 2012, pp. 296–301. doi:10.3945/ajcn.112.035782.

42. Ohkawara, Kazunori, et al. "Effects of Increased Meal Frequency on Fat Oxidation and Perceived Hunger." *Obesity*, vol. 21, no. 2, 2013, pp. 336–343. doi:10.1002/oby.20032.

43. Patel, J. N. "Norepinephrine Spillover from Human Adipose Tissue before and after a 72-Hour Fast." *Journal of Clinical Endocrinology & Metabolism*, vol. 87, no. 7, Jan. 2002, pp. 3373–3377. doi:10.1210/jc.87.7.3373.

44. Popkin, Barry M., et al. "Water, Hydration, and Health." *Nutrition Reviews*, vol. 68, no. 8, Aug. 2010, pp. 439-458. doi:10.1111/j.1753-4887.2010.00304.x.

45. Quiclet, Charline, et al. "Pancreatic Adipocytes Mediate Hypersecretion of Insulin in Diabetes-Susceptible Mice." *Metabolism*, vol. 97, 2019, pp. 9–17. doi:10.1016/j.metabol.2019.05.005.

46. Rakicioglu, Neslisah, et al. "The Effect of Ramadan on Maternal Nutrition and Composition of Breast Milk." *Pediatrics International*, vol. 48, no. 3, 2006, pp. 278–283. doi:10.1111/j.1442-200x.2006.02204.x.

47. Reed, Eric. "What Is the Average Household Cost of Food in 2019?" *The Street*, 25 Jan. 2019, https://www.thestreet.com/personal-finance/average-cost-of-food-14845479.

48. "Reversing Type 2 Diabetes in Only 2.5 Months with Keto and Fasting." *Diet Doctor*, 3 Jan. 2019,

https://www.dietdoctor.com/reversing-type-2-diabetes-1-5-months-Keto-fasting.

49. Rosenbaum, M., and R. L. Leibel. "Adaptive Thermogenesis in Humans." *International Journal of Obesity*, vol. 34, 2010, pp. S47-S55. doi:10.1038/ijo.2010.184.

50. Runcie, J., and T. J. Thomson. "Prolonged Starvation-A Dangerous Procedure." *British Medical Journal*, vol. 3, no. 432, 22 Aug. 1970. doi:10.1136/bmj.3.5720.432.

51. Schoenfeld, B. Jon, et al. "Effects of Meal Frequency on Weight Loss and Body Composition: a Meta-Analysis." *Nutrition Reviews*, vol. 73, no. 2, 2015, pp. 69–82. doi:10.1093/nutrit/nuu017.

52. Seimon, Radhika V., et al. "Do Intermittent Diets Provide Physiological Benefits over Continuous Diets for Weight Loss? A Systematic Review of Clinical Trials." *Molecular and Cellular Endocrinology*, vol. 418, 2015, pp. 153–172. doi:10.1016/j.mce.2015.09.014.

53. Simmons, D., et al. "The New Zealand Diabetes Passport Study: a Randomized Controlled Trial of the Impact of a Diabetes Passport on Risk Factors for Diabetes-Related Complications." *Diabetic Medicine*, vol. 21, no. 3, 2004, pp. 214–217. doi:10.1111/j.1464-5491.2004.01047.x.

54. Smeets, Astrid J., and Margriet S. Westerterp-Plantenga. "Acute Effects on Metabolism and Appetite Profile of One Meal Difference in the Lower Range of Meal Frequency." *British Journal of*

Nutrition, vol. 99, no. 6, 2008, pp. 1316–1321. doi:10.1017/s0007114507877646.

55. Speechly, D.p., and R. Buffenstein. "Greater Appetite Control Associated with an Increased Frequency of Eating in Lean Males." *Appetite*, vol. 33, no. 3, 1999, pp. 285–297. doi:10.1006/appe.1999.0265.

56. St-Pierre, Valérie, et al. "Plasma Ketone and Medium Chain Fatty Acid Response in Humans Consuming Different Medium Chain Triglycerides During a Metabolic Study Day." *Frontiers in Nutrition*, vol. 6, 2019. doi:10.3389/fnut.2019.00046.

57. Siegel, Rebecca L., et al. "Cancer Statistics, 2019." *CA: A Cancer Journal for Clinicians*, vol. 69, no. 1, 8 Jan. 2019. doi:10.3322/caac.21551.

58. "Success Stories." *Gin Stephens, Author and Intermittent Faster*, http://www.ginstephens.com/success-stories.html.

59. Sutton, Elizabeth F., et al. "Early Time-Restricted Feeding Improves Insulin Sensitivity, Blood Pressure, and Oxidative Stress Even without Weight Loss in Men with Prediabetes." *Cell Metabolism*, vol. 27, no. 6, 2018. doi:10.1016/j.cmet.2018.04.010.

60. Trepanowski, John F., et al. "Effect of Alternate-Day Fasting on Weight Loss, Weight Maintenance, and Cardioprotection Among Metabolically Healthy Obese Adults." *JAMA Internal Medicine*, vol. 177, no. 7, Jan. 2017, p. 930. doi:10.1001/jamainternmed.2017.0936.

61. Varady, K. A. "Intermittent versus Daily Calorie Restriction: Which Diet Regimen Is More Effective

for Weight Loss?" Obesity Reviews, vol. 12, no. 7, 2011, doi:10.1111/j.1467-789x.2011.00873.x.

62. Vasconcelos, Andrea Rodrigues, et al. "Effects of Intermittent Fasting on Age-Related Changes on Na,K-ATPase Activity and Oxidative Status Induced by Lipopolysaccharide in Rat Hippocampus." *Neurobiology of Aging*, vol. 36, no. 5, 2015, pp. 1914–1923. doi:10.1016/j.neurobiolaging.2015.02.020.

63. Watkins, Ellen, and Lucy Serpell. "The Psychological Effects of Short-Term Fasting in Healthy Women." *Frontiers in Nutrition*, vol. 3, no. 27, 22 Aug. 2016. doi:10.3389/fnut.2016.00027

64. Webb, Sherrie R. "AHA 2019 Heart Disease and Stroke Statistics." *American College of Cardiology,* https://www.acc.org/latest-in-cardiology/ten-points-to-remember/2019/02/15/14/39/aha-2019-heart-disease-and-stroke-statistics.

65. Weigle, David S., et al. "High-Protein Diet Induces Sustained Reductions in Appetite, Ad Libitum Caloric Intake, and Body Weight despite Compensatory Changes in Diurnal Plasma Leptin and Ghrelin Concentrations." *The American Journal of Clinical Nutrition*, vol. 82, no. 1, 1 July 2005, pp. 41-48. doi:10.1093/ajcn/82.1.41

66. Zauner, Christian, et al. "Resting Energy Expenditure in Short-Term Starvation Is Increased as a Result of an Increase in Serum Norepinephrine." *The American Journal of Clinical Nutrition*, vol. 71, no. 6, Jan. 2000, pp. 1511–1515., doi:10.1093/ajcn/71.6.1511.

www.ingramcontent.com/pod-product-compliance
Lightning Source LLC
Chambersburg PA
CBHW061758250726
48657CB00001B/189